COUPLE THERAPY FOR ALCOHOLISM

THE GUILFORD SUBSTANCE ABUSE SERIES
Howard T. Blane and Thomas R. Kosten, *Editors*

Recent Volumes

COUPLE THERAPY FOR ALCOHOLISM

A Cognitive-Behavioral Treatment Manual

Phylis J. Wakefield
Rebecca E. Williams
Elizabeth B. Yost
Kathleen M. Patterson

Foreword by
Larry E. Beutler
Theodore Jacob
Varda Shoham

THE GUILFORD PRESS
New York   London

©1996 The Guilford Press
A Division of Guilford Publications, Inc.
72 Spring Street, New York, NY 10012

Printed in the United States of America

This book is printed on acid-free paper.

Last digit is print number: 9 8 7 6 5 4 3 2 1

Library of Congress Cataloging-in-Publication Data

Couple therapy for alcoholism : a cognitive-behavioral treatment
manual / by Phylis J. Wakefield . . . [et al.].
    p.   cm.—(The Guilford substance abuse series)
  Includes bibliographical references and index.
  ISBN 1–57230–070–1
  1. Alcoholism—Treatment. 2. Marital psychotherapy. 3. Cognitive
therapy. I. Wakefield, Phylis J. II. Series.
  [DNLM: 1. Alcoholism—therapy. 2. Marital Therapy—methods.
3. Cognitive Therapy. WM 274 C857 1996]
  RC565.C598   1996
  616.86'10651—dc20
  DNLM/DLC   95-40825
                                                              CIP

To Dr. Larry E. Beutler,
for his unyielding commitment
to our professional development

Acknowledgments

Phylis J. Wakefield would like to thank her husband, Andre, for his support and encouragement throughout this project.

Rebecca E. Williams would like to thank her family, Joan, Herbert, and Rachel for such a strong foundation on which to build. She would also like to thank Julie Meisels and Laura Forsyth for their enduring friendships.

Elizabeth B. Yost would like to thank Jody.

Kathleen M. Patterson would like to thank her children, Jesse and Lara, for their love and patience.

The authors would also like to thank Stephanie Entwistle, a very dedicated undergraduate research assistant, for her help during critical moments of this project.

Foreword

This book was conceived from a continuing research program that the three of us (Larry E. Beutler, Theodore Jacob, and Varda Shoham) developed and initiated in 1990. Dr. Elizabeth Yost is a coinvestigator on that project and the coordinator of the effort that resulted in the cognitive therapy protocol described here. Phylis J. Wakefield, Rebecca E. Williams, and Kathleen M. Patterson were extraordinarily gifted graduate students who became members of Liz's team. Together this group assumed the responsibility for describing and then applying the principles of cognitive therapy to alcoholic couples.

The history of this book is intimately tied to the larger history of the research project from which it derives. The project was born of a long-standing friendship between two of us (Beutler and Jacob), dating back to the late 1960s when we both were graduate students at the University of Nebraska. In the mid-1980s we became colleagues at the University of Arizona and shortly thereafter were joined by Varda Shoham, who initially accepted a visiting professorship with Beutler. Later, Shoham assumed a full-time faculty position, and the three of us began to explore ways in which Jacob's interest in alcoholic family interactional styles, Beutler's interest in differential psychotherapy efficacy, and Shoham's interests in system's therapy and psychotherapy research could be linked in a potentially productive fashion.

Beginning in the fall of 1987, acting as Co-Principal Investigators, we began exploring our research interests through a series of early Monday morning meetings. As our plans were clarified, it became apparent that the diversity of our interests was energizing. The evolving research program earned funding approval from the National Institute on Alcohol Abuse and Alcoholism (Grant No. RO1-AA08970) in 1990 as Beutler was in the process of moving to the University of California–Santa Barbara (UCSB).

The focus of the research program from which this book is derived has been to develop and test two treatments for alcoholic men and women. This book represents a manualized intervention that incorporates behavioral strategies; the other treatment involves a manualized, family systems intervention for alcoholism. The objectives that the larger research program was designed to accomplish evolved from an awareness that, in spite of the progress that has been made in the development and application of effective treatment interventions for alcoholism, empirical comparisons have found no one treatment approach to be consistently superior to any other. Indeed, research literature has largely failed to identify reliable differences between residential (usually a standard 28-day inpatient program) and nonresidential treatment settings, or between long-term and short-term interventions. We came to believe that differential treatment effects would become evident only when aspects of the patient's functional behavior beyond those reflected in the diagnosis of alcohol dependence were considered. This conclusion was similar to those that were simultaneously emerging from those who studied depression, anxiety, and other mental and behavioral disorders.

As we planned this project, our combined wisdom led us to believe that at least two distinctly different alcoholism subtypes exist—one characterized by an episodic style of drinking, high levels of social impairment, and greater hostile, externalizing, and antisocial tendencies; the other characterized by a more continuous style of drinking, less social impairment, and possibly passive and unassertive tendencies. Interestingly, Jacob's research had indicated that these two types of alcoholics established quite different marriages, the former characterized by negativity and coercion and the latter by increased stability associated with periods of heavy drinking.

Inspection of the general psychotherapy literature indicated illuminating parallels between these alcoholism subtypes and subtypes of psychotherapy patients with nonalcoholic psychopathologies. We came to believe that diversified treatment approaches may be differentially useful for various patient types, a point of view for which we found some support in research literature across a variety of patient groups. Previous work by Beutler distinguishing between "externalizing" and "internalizing" coping styles revealed conceptual similarities to Jacob's contrast between "episodic" and "steady" drinkers.

We also came to appreciate the distinctions made by Peter Steinglass between families with an alcoholic member and "alcoholic families."

Based on these observations, we hypothesized that those alcoholics with externalizing and internalizing coping styles may benefit from different types of treatment. Our research program and this book are devoted to that proposition. We believe that among externalizing, impulsive alcoholic patients, the direct treatment of behavioral patterns described in this volume might be most advantageous, with improved family patterns accompanying and reflecting the improvement but not causing it.

The research project to which this book contributes continues, now as a joint venture among the University of California (Beutler), where the project is administered and the treatment trials are conducted; the University of Arizona (Shoham), where the psychotherapy process measures are analyzed and the family systems therapy is monitored; and the Palo Alto Department of Veterans Affairs Medical Center (Jacob), where the family/couple interaction data are evaluated. At this time, we have only preliminary results on the efficacy of the couple therapy (covered in this volume) and the family systems therapy studied in this project. Complete analysis of that data will be forthcoming and will be published through the usual peer review process.

Through good fortune and some planning, our research group was joined early on by a variety of productive, congenial, and stimulating scholars who have served as coinvestigators, therapists, consultants, colleagues, supervisors, and coordinators. Among the most significant of these, of course, are the authors of this book. Elizabeth B. Yost has been an especially valued colleague and coinvestigator. She has worked for many years with Beutler and this is the second manual on cognitive therapy that she has developed out of this collaboration. Her continuing contributions and dedication are very much appreciated by all of us.

The couple therapy work also has benefited immeasurably from interactions with our colleagues who helped to develop the family systems treatment manual, the major comparison treatment in our project. These colleagues include Michael Rohrbaugh, Peter Steinglass, and Carol Spungen. The cognitive therapists, who were willingly trained and have enthusiastically tolerated the demands of the research protocol in order to implement this manual, have been Phylis J. Wakefield, Rebecca E. Williams, Andy Winzelberg, Stuart Light, Sherry Hummel, Melinda McCain Dale, Alison Hubbard, Mitch Karno, and Mark Harwood. The family systems therapists have included Carol Spungen, Lael Foster, Barbara Sheffield, Tracey St. Johns, Andres Consoli, Vicki Matica, Estella Escoboza, Robert Schreiber, and Carol Crump. We thank them all for their devotion and patience.

Many other colleagues, graduate students, and friends have assisted in the overall project, among the most notable of whom have been Barbara McCrady, Timothy O'Farrell, and Neil Jacobson, all of whom served as consultants during the development of these ideas. Additionally, Drs. Jasna Jovanovic and Heidi Zetzer served, at various stages, as project coordinators, and Lynn Peterson was immensely helpful as the administrative assistant and support staff for the Principal Investigator (Beutler). We also acknowledge the personal support of many other past and current students; the GSE Research Office staff at UCSB; and the family systems therapists and the research teams at UCSB, the University of Arizona, Palo Alto Department of Veterans Affairs Medical Center, and the College of William and Mary. The contributions of all of these people are reflected in our work but are too numerous to mention. To this long list, we add the colleagues and friends who are numbered within our professional reference groups, particularly the Society for Psychotherapy Research, both the North American and International organizations. Without the tireless efforts of these and others, this production would have been significantly limited. Most of all, we appreciate the work of the authors of this manual for taking our loose images and hypotheses and defining them in concrete and specific terms.

LARRY E. BEUTLER
THEODORE JACOB
VARDA SHOHAM

Contents

ACUTE PHASE

RELAPSE PREVENTION PHASE

TERMINATION PHASE

APPENDICES

FORMS

CHAPTER 1

Introduction

Given the pervasiveness of alcohol problems in this country, there is a pressing need for treatment that is both brief and effective. The Institute of Medicine (IOM, 1990) reviewed over 600 outcome studies in the field of alcohol treatment and concluded that, although no one treatment approach works for all individuals with alcohol problems, the provision of appropriate, specific treatment modalities can improve outcome. Such treatment has proven to be more effective when it is oriented toward ongoing life circumstances and when it addresses attendant life problems through the inclusion of such techniques as social skills training, marital therapy, and stress management (IOM, 1990).

In the past few years, a number of books have been published that address this need from a cognitive-behavioral perspective. Inpatient/outpatient group training in socials skills has been outlined by Monti and his colleagues (Monti, Abrams, Kadden, & Cooney, 1989). Beck's group (Beck, Wright, Newman, & Liese, 1993) has offered a manual of cognitive therapy for alcoholism and other addictions. The Sobells (1993) have published a self-help book for treating the alcohol-related life problems of problem drinkers. The theoretical and empirical basis for couple treatment for alcoholism has been presented by O'Farrell (1993). As a complement to these works, our book presents a model for time-limited, cognitive-behavioral outpatient treatment for alcoholism within the context of couple therapy.

We have based our treatment on the behavioral premise that alcoholism is learned behavior that is reinforced and maintained from a variety of sources. Alcoholics can learn to identify the internal and external cues that lead them to drink. They can also learn to use their own cognitions and behavioral resources as well as the support of other people to cope with these situations. The role of the therapist in this approach is one of

an educator and a consultant who teaches alcoholic clients the intrapersonal and interpersonal coping skills needed to live without alcohol.

To this end, the alcoholic is instructed in strategies to achieve and
maintain abstinence. Alcohol-related life problems, such as relationship
concerns and social skills deficits, are also addressed. Partners of the
alcoholics participate fully in all stages of the treatment by learning about
the ways in which their behavior may serve as cues and reinforcers for the
alcoholic's drinking or cues and reinforcers for abstinence. Partners also
choose a behavior of their own that they wish to decrease or eliminate,
thereby engaging in a process parallel to that of the alcoholic.

In this introductory chapter, we briefly review the behavioral perspective on alcoholism and present the theoretical and empirical support for
treating alcoholics in a couple context. The rationale for having the
partner engage in a process that parallels that of the alcoholic is explained,
and suggestions for the implementation of treatment are offered.

BEHAVIORAL VIEW OF ALCOHOLISM

From a behavioral or social learning perspective, alcoholism is a biopsy-
chosocial process, the course of which is determined by multiple factors
(Abrams, 1983). According to this model, alcoholism and other addictive
behaviors are habitual, maladaptive methods for attempting to cope with
the stresses of daily living. Although genetic or biological vulnerability
may predispose a given individual to drink excessively in response to
stress, the conditions for drinking are determined by that person's social
learning history. What, where, when, and how drinking occurs, as well as
attitudes and expectancies toward drinking, are all learned. The combination of alcoholics' genetic vulnerability coupled with their social learning history generally results in multiple deficits in social skills (Monti et
al., 1989). Not only do alcoholics tend to overrely on alcohol as a way to
cope with life stresses, they also fail to develop other coping skills as a
consequence of this reliance on alcohol. The focus of treatment for
alcoholics, then, is twofold. Not only must they unlearn drinking behavior,
they must also replace it by learning more adaptive methods for coping
with stress.

In recent years, there has been much controversy over whether
alcoholism is a disease. Given the numerous ways in which the learning
environment affects the development and the treatment of alcoholism, the
question of whether alcoholism is a disease may be of less importance for
treatment than the concept of helping alcoholics learn about their drinking
behavior in order to change it. Indeed, Morgenstern and McCrady (1992),
in their review of the alcohol and drug literature, noted that there has been

a movement toward the integration of behavioral treatment processes into the traditional disease model.

FACTORS THAT AFFECT DRINKING BEHAVIOR

Monti and his colleagues (1989), in their coping skills manual for the treatment of alcoholics, delineated the ways in which drinking behavior is influenced by cognitive-behavioral principles and by social learning history. The specific principles of reinforcement, conditioning, cognitions and expectancy, self-efficacy, and social modeling are briefly reviewed to provide a foundation for this manual.

First and foremost, alcohol use is both *positively and negatively reinforcing* in a variety of ways (Monti et al., 1989). The principle of positive reinforcement states that the likelihood of a behavior being repeated is increased when it is followed by a pleasant consequence. The physiological sensations of warmth and relaxation produced by the effects of alcohol are extremely pleasurable, and therefore positively reinforcing to many people. On an interpersonal level, alcohol consumption may be positively reinforced by providing increased feelings of social confidence and conviviality. The principle of negative reinforcement states that the likelihood of a behavior being repeated is increased when it is followed by the removal of an unpleasant consequence. The sensations of warmth and relaxation produced by the ingestion of alcohol may lead to a reduction of tension, loneliness, sadness, or other feeling states that are often considered aversive. Through this release of tension, alcohol use is negatively reinforcing. Indeed, individuals with problems of alcohol abuse may know of no other ways to reduce unpleasant affect. On an interpersonal level, negative reinforcement may come from the reduction of the sensations of awkwardness and discomfort in social situations. It is useful for the therapist to be aware that the alcoholic is likely to suffer significant feelings of loss when a substance that is reinforcing in so many ways is removed. During treatment, alternative behaviors that are reinforcing by supplying pleasure and by reducing pain must be found to replace alcohol.

According to the principles of *classical conditioning*, previously neutral events gain strength through frequent association to a stimulus that is naturally potent. As previously noted, alcohol use is highly reinforcing. Therefore, it may readily become associated by principles of classical conditioning to stimuli both in the immediate, personal environment and in the more distant, impersonal environment (Monti et al., 1989). Any person, place, or thing that has been frequently associated with alcohol consumption in the past can serve as a stimulus or cue that prompts drinking in the present. Cues in the interpersonal environment may be watching a sporting event on television, driving past a favorite bar, or attending a social event at which drinking is the norm. Cues in the personal environment may be a partner's tone of voice, a family dispute, or a family gathering where alcohol is always served. The likelihood of alcohol consumption can be decreased by the use of stimulus control, which minimizes the exposure to cues that promote drinking. It may be relatively easier for alcoholics to practice stimulus control by avoiding cues in the interpersonal environment than it would be to make changes in their personal environment. For example, one can more readily change one's route home from work or turn off a beer commercial on television than one can change the behavior of one's spouse or parents. However, changes in the personal environment are needed in order for changes in drinking behavior to be maintained (Bandura, 1977a).

Cognitive distortions and expectancies (Beck, Rush, Shaw, & Emery, 1979) also play a role in maintaining drinking behavior. Urges to drink are often accompanied by irrational beliefs and expectations. For example, the belief that one needs a drink to get through a particularly difficult situation is an irrational belief that may exacerbate alcohol consumption. The prospect of attending a family gathering or an office party without drinking may feel overwhelming to alcoholics. They may firmly believe that it is impossible for them to survive in such situations without using alcohol. They may say to themselves such things as, "I can't face this event sober. I can't get through this evening without a drink." In treatment, these irrational cognitions need to be identified and more rational, adaptive self-statements substituted in their place.

Drinking behavior, particularly the possibility of relapsing from sobriety (Marlatt & Gordon, 1985), is further affected by the alcoholic's sense of *self-efficacy* (Bandura, 1977a). Self-efficacy is one's sense of confidence and ability to master difficult or challenging situations. According to this model, when alcoholics face high-risk situations and are able to cope successfully they experience an increased sense of self-efficacy, which leads to a decreased likelihood of relapse. Conversely, the lack of successful coping responses leads to a feeling of decreased self-efficacy and the increased probability of relapse. Teaching alcoholics alternative coping responses in therapy augments their sense of self-efficacy and reduces chances of relapse.

Social expectancies and rules for drinking behavior are culturally transmitted by *modeling* (Bandura, 1977b) in the family, in the media, and in the social interactions of peers (Monti et al., 1989). Parents model any number of drinking habits for their children; for example, they may model that drinking is forbidden or, conversely, that a drink is needed to help one relax after work. Peers model the behavior that is required in order to be accepted as part of the group. Commercial advertisements not only impart information about specific products, but also transmit information about drinking styles. From a treatment perspective, it is important to be aware of the ways in which clients understand the place of drinking in society in general, as well as in their own lives. In addition, it is important to help them find opportunities to observe alternative behaviors both within and outside of the treatment session.

In summary, according to cognitive-behavioral and social learning theory, alcoholism is a process that is reinforced by multiple interpersonal as well as intrapersonal factors. Monti and colleagues (1989) found that alcoholics who were taught interpersonal coping skills improved most, not only in alcohol relevant skills but also in relaxation and mood management. That is, training in social skills increased the alcoholics' facility with intrapersonal skills as well. Furthermore, research has found that relapse from abstinence can be predicted by both intrapersonal and interpersonal processes (Cummings, Gordon, & Marlatt, 1980). The alcoholics' primary relationship provides an excellent context in which to teach social skills. It is also the context in which these skills might most often be needed and utilized if abstinence is to be maintained.

COUPLE TREATMENT FOR ALCOHOLISM

One of the most influential sources of interpersonal reinforcement, including reinforcement of drinking behavior, is the family (Gondoli & Jacob, 1990). As we have seen, drinking behavior is difficult to eliminate because it is inextricably bound to daily routines and interactions, many of which take place in the home. The behavior of each partner in a marital relationship can serve as either a cue or a reinforcer for the other's behavior. This means that the partner can also promote those changes in the alcoholic's everyday environment that are necessary to maintain changes in drinking behavior (McCrady et al., 1986).

Clinical and research evidence supports the reciprocal relationship between conflicted marital and family interactions and abusive drinking. O'Farrell (1989) found that marital conflicts are frequently precipitators to relapse. There is a higher incidence of marital discord, divorce, separation, and child and spousal abuse in families in which there is abusive drinking (O'Farrell, 1989; O'Farrell & Murphy, 1995). Longabaugh, Beattie, Stout, Malloy, and Noel (1988) found that for individuals highly invested in their social environment there was a strong relationship between the amount of support for sobriety tendered by this environment and the proportion of days abstinent in the year following treatment. However, this was not the case for persons not similarly invested.

Applying a relapse prevention model to couple treatment, McCrady

(1989) noted that alcoholic coping responses are affected by (1) the quality of the social support network, (2) the quality of the primary intimate relationship, (3) the density of reinforcement for abstinence, and (4) a lack of reinforcement for drinking. When these factors are considered, it becomes apparent that partners are in a position to be highly influential in helping or hindering alcoholics in their efforts to maintain abstinence. Partners have the potential to serve as an invaluable source of social support for the alcoholics as they attempt to change drinking behavior and to maintain those changes over time (Jacobson, Holtzworth-Munroe, & Schmaling, 1989). Furthermore, the partner's response to the alcoholic may help either to prevent or to encourage relapse.

In our experience, partners of the alcoholics are often more desirous of change, and therefore more motivated to enter treatment, than the alcoholics themselves. Offering couple therapy provides a legitimate avenue of action for partners who are concerned about their alcoholics' drinking problems. Nonalcoholic partners frequently are the ones who initiate treatment and, at least initially, may be more committed to attending sessions than the alcoholics themselves.

Spouse-Involved Cognitive-Behavioral Therapy

Spouse-involved cognitive-behavioral therapy provides training to the alcoholics both in the intrapersonal skills needed to attain abstinence and in the interpersonal skills needed to improve their functioning in the social sphere. On an intrapersonal level, the alcoholics learn techniques to facilitate the maintenance of abstinence, such as stimulus control and rational self-statements. On an interpersonal level, problems within the marriage, the workplace, and the broader social support network are all addressed. Although not as widely used in treatment settings as either family systems therapy or therapy based upon a disease model of alcoholism, spouse-involved cognitive-behavioral treatment has been well researched in controlled outcome studies (Gondoli & Jacob, 1990).

Research has found (O'Farrell, 1991) that behavioral couple therapy for alcoholism can (1) provide the motivation necessary for making the initial commitment to change and for continuing in treatment on the part of the alcoholic, (2) stabilize both the marital relationship and abstinent behavior 1 year posttreatment, and (3) reduce the deterioration of, and support the maintenance of, gains in the marital relationship and drinking behavior in the long term. A 2-year follow-up study (O'Farrell, Cutter, Choquette, & Bayog, 1992) that compared couples who received behavioral marital therapy (BMT) in addition to alcohol counseling to those who received no marital therapy found better marital outcomes for the BMT group. Specifically, the wives (but not the husbands) evidenced better marital adjustment and there were fewer separation days during the 2-year period. These results did, however, seem to fade over time. In terms of drinking outcomes, the superiority of the addition of BMT was not apparent at the end of 2 years, even though this effect had been noted at the end of treatment.

McCrady and her colleagues (1986) compared the treatment of alcoholics and their spouses under three conditions: (1) minimal spouse involvement, (2) alcohol-focused spouse involvement, and (3) alcohol-focused spouse involvement plus BMT. They found that spouses in the minimal involvement group dropped out of treatment more frequently than spouses in the other groups. The participants in the BMT group were more compliant with conjoint homework assignments and showed a higher level of marital satisfaction. At 18-month follow-up, this higher level of marital satisfaction continued and participants reported fewer marital separations. In addition, the alcoholics in this group tended to decrease drinking more quickly after entering treatment and showed greater maintenance of treatment gains at 6- and 18-month follow-up. The conclusion of this study indicated that involvement of spouses improves outcome for the alcoholics, but that the *spouses must be motivated to remain in treatment by addressing issues that are important to them beyond the problems of the alcoholics.*

The Parallel Process of the Partner

In this book, the partners' work to decrease or eliminate a specific targeted behavior is designed to increase the partners' motivation to remain in treatment. To this end, the partners complete the same in-session and out-of-session exercises as the alcoholics. The focus of these exercises is the partners' chosen target behavior (e.g., overeating, overspending, smoking) rather than alcohol use. In instances where both individuals are problem drinkers, the partner may choose alcohol as a target behavior to eliminate (see Chapter 3 for a discussion of both members of the couple having a drinking problem).

A further reason to engage the partners in a parallel process is that they often come into treatment with a backlog of years of anger and resentment. Having a project of their own to focus on during treatment can provide an avenue for the partners to redirect their energy away from reactions to the alcoholic toward helping themselves. Indeed, even though it is important for the therapist to acknowledge the partner's intense emotions in relation to the alcoholic, it is often not possible or advisable to spend a great deal of time in session addressing these emotions directly. Giving the partners a positive, personal place in the treatment program may reduce the chance that they will sabotage treatment by continually attempting to draw the therapist's attention to their feelings of anger and resentment. Frequently, alcohol-conflicted couples are locked into a non-productive cycle of mutual blame and recrimination. When both members of the couple have issues to address independently, this cycle of blaming may be interrupted. The partners' project provides a means by which the focus can shift from worrying about the alcoholics' drinking to highlighting and exploring their own problems. This approach may also offer partners a way to experience changing behaviors that are within their power and capability to change.

When both members of the couple are engaged in a similar process, the couple becomes a small group in which each member can model successful coping strategies for the other. Furthermore, working in a parallel process can increase the ability of either partner to empathize with the struggles of the other in relinquishing a well-entrenched habit. The partner is likely to experience both successes and setbacks when attending to his or her own targeted behavior. This will provide a rich framework for the partner to understand the successes and setbacks of the alcoholic as well as for the alcoholic to sympathize with the successes and setbacks of his or her partner.

IMPLEMENTATION OF THIS MANUAL

This manual is designed primarily for use with outpatients with a primary diagnosis of alcohol abuse or dependence (American Psychiatric Association, 1994) who have already been through the process of detoxification or for whom detoxification is not indicated. As such, it is useful for the treatment of individuals whose insurance will pay for a few days of inpatient detoxification and brief outpatient treatment. Research has found (W. R. Miller & Hester, 1986) that there is no difference in effectiveness in outpatient and inpatient treatment for alcoholism. Indeed, the exercises presented in this book are best implemented if the alcoholics and their partners are following their normal daily routines as much as possible. Outpatient treatment allows the alcoholics to confront those situations of daily life in which they usually drink and provides an opportunity for them to attempt to abstain from drinking. Any successes that they experience in coping with stressful situations without drinking can be reinforced in subsequent therapy sessions. The more numerous and various the situations in which they are successful in abstaining from alcohol, the greater the likelihood of generalization of nondrinking behavior to other situations that will arise in the future. In addition, "lapses," a single occurrence of drinking while trying to maintain abstinence (Marlatt & Gordon, 1985), can be discussed within the therapy hour as situations from which to learn, rather than as predictors of failure.

The treatment approach presented in this book would also be suitable for couples seeking counseling for whom alcohol abuse is a problem that they may not yet have clearly identified and/or acknowledged. Such couples generally know that something is wrong with their relationship but they cannot quite identify what it is. If alcohol abuse is an area that one partner mentions as a problem, this program, which focuses on both alcoholism and the relationship, may be suggested as a treatment option.

Abstinence as a Treatment Goal

It should be noted that in this treatment model, abstinence, not controlled drinking, is advocated as the goal of treatment. Controlled and/or moderated drinking approaches are generally not advised for clients with a history of severe physical dependence on alcohol (Rosenberg, 1993). Data suggest that such an approaches are both ineffectual and unethical as treatment goals for chronic alcoholics (Nathan, 1986). Abstinence as a goal of treatment is consistent with the current standards of practice in the field.

Although this book focuses primarily on abstinence from alcohol and the language herein is consistent with this focus, the goal of treatment is for clients to be abstinent from all other psychoactive drugs. If clients continue to use other drugs, even though they are abstaining from alcohol, treatment will be hampered and the probability of relapse will increase. The new coping skills introduced in treatment, if learned while under the influence of any psychoactive substance, will more readily generalize to an intoxicated state than to a sober state. Therefore, it is important to ask the alcoholics and their partners routinely if they have used or are continuing to use other drugs. If they are using other drugs, discuss with them the inadvisability of doing so while in treatment for alcohol abuse.

12-STEP PROGRAMS

This chapter would not be complete without mention of clients' participation in Alcoholics Anonymous (AA), which has been cited as the most frequently prescribed treatment for alcohol-dependent individuals (Beutler, Jovanovic, & Williams, 1993). Clients who have previous or current involvement in AA may have difficulty reconciling the cognitive-behavioral approach with the 12-step approach. The first two steps, which require that alcoholics acknowledge that they are powerless over alcohol and that they turn their problems over to a Higher Power, may be particularly problematic. The language used in this book, which encourages empowerment by teaching clients ways to control situations in which they are tempted to drink, may seem to some clients to contradict the first two steps. However, we have found that the cognitive-behavioral approach may easily be framed as a complement to a 12-step program. It may be helpful to point out to clients who attend AA that, although they may be powerless over alcohol, they are *not* powerless over sobriety or other areas of their lives. Turning their problems with alcohol over to a Higher Power does not preclude the possibility of learning new skills and behaviors to enhance their lives. We believe that the goal of this treatment program, which is to teach the alcoholic new cognitions and behaviors to help maintain sobriety, is not incompatible with the goals of AA. The AA slogan "identify, don't compare" may be used to help clients recognize that they may choose whatever elements they find useful from either approach. It does not make sense to attempt to compare cognitive-behavioral treatment and AA as each involves different strategies and techniques. However, both this program and the AA model recommend abstinence from alcohol as an aim for healthier living.

Al-Anon, a self-help program designed for partners and family members of alcoholics, may also be a positive adjunct for the partners of the alcoholics who have decided on couple therapy as their treatment of choice. Although research in the area of multiple addiction and use of anonymous groups is scarce, some alcoholics who are also struggling with other drug dependencies may be well served by attending AA and other anonymous groups such as Narcotics Anonymous (NA) or Cocaine Anonymous (CA).

Partners who have chosen an addictive behavior, such as smoking, as a target for treatment may benefit from attending an anonymous group geared to eliminating that behavior, such as Smokers Anonymous. Essentially, accessing support during and after treatment is a good indication of high client motivation not only to address problem behavior but also to incorporate these changes in overall lifestyle.

THE ORGANIZATION OF THIS MANUAL

The treatment approach outlined in this book is based on a 20-session model, although the material in each chapter may stand alone and be integrated into a variety of other therapeutic approaches. We present five phases of treatment (Preparation, Early Treatment, Middle Treatment, Relapse Prevention, and End of Treatment) and offer recommendations on how many sessions should be spent on each of these phases of treatment. If using the 20-session model, a sample meeting schedule may be found in Appendix 1.

In each phase of treatment, the amount and type of information presented reflects the differential ability of alcoholics to use and retain information throughout the process of recovery. Simple skills are taught initially because early in treatment the alcoholic may be unable to process cognitively complex material (Monti et al., 1989). More difficult tasks, building upon previously learned skills, are introduced in later sessions when the alcoholic may be better able to process more complex information. Early sessions of therapy focus on establishing the therapeutic relationship, on increasing the clients' motivation, and on enhancing the clients' compliance with out-of-session exercises. In the middle sessions of therapy, the therapist focuses on teaching the skills and strategies needed to achieve and maintain abstinence and to enhance the couple relationship. In the final sessions, the focus of treatment is on formulating a specific relapse prevention plan, on establishing a nondrinking social support network, and on addressing other alcohol-related life problems, such as poor nutrition, excessive smoking, lack of exercise, inadequate sleep, difficulties in sexual behavior, development of relaxation, and satisfaction in the work environment.

Chapter 1 has provided you with an overview of the general philosophy underlying the treatment approach introduced in this book as well as introducing important treatment considerations when working with alcoholic-conflicted couples.

Chapter 2 focuses on the special considerations of women alcoholics and includes the following topics: drinking and help-seeking behavior, psychiatric history and current life stressors, physiological vulnerability to the effects of alcohol, reproductive complications, marital and family functioning and parenting, domestic violence, cultural factors, and treatment considerations for women.

Chapter 3 outlines the Preparation Phase of treatment. The topics of the chapter include (1) building rapport with clients, (2) gathering relevant psychological and substance abuse history, (3) preparing clients for therapy, (4) agreeing on therapeutic goals, and (5) deciding on the time and frequency of sessions. Also discussed in the chapter are four general therapist expectations that provide a framework for discussing the cognitive-behavioral approach to treating alcoholism, the advantages of treating the alcoholic in the context of a couple, the expectation of abstinence as a primary goal, and the active participation of the partner in a treatment process parallel to that of the alcoholic client. The Preparation Phase concludes with the formulation of a Behavioral Contract that outlines the therapeutic goals and provides a bridge into the Early Treatment Phase.

Chapter 4 outlines the Early Treatment Phase, inclusive of the following goals: (1) engaging the couple in treatment, (2) teaching self-monitoring and exploring the clients' triggers for drinking and the target behavior, and (3) introducing the concept of "pleasant events" to enhance the couple's relationship in early abstinence. The self-monitoring charts, called the Drinking Chain I and Target Behavior Chart I, are introduced in this phase of treatment. Alcoholic clients are asked to monitor cravings and thoughts about drinking, and partners are asked to monitor cravings and thoughts about their targeted behavior. These charts are a central therapeutic tool used throughout the treatment program.

Chapter 5, the introduction of the communication skills training, serves as an adjunct to the Early and Middle Treatment Phases. The goals of this chapter include teaching clients (1) how to express thoughts and feelings clearly and assertively, (2) effective listening skills, (3) how to give each other positive reinforcement, and (4) how to give each other feedback. These communication skills are presented in a graded manner with easier skills appearing first, followed by more advanced skills. Level I communication skills include "I" messages, perception checks, and positive reinforcement. Level II communication skills include reflective listening and attending. Level III communication skills include giving and receiving feedback. Incorporating these skills into treatment as early as possible, and providing time to practice them often, will enhance the clients' relationship and help create a more supportive environment for recovery.

Chapter 6 outlines the Middle Treatment Phase. The strategies and the goals include (1) teaching more complex self-monitoring skills, (2) teaching cognitive and behavioral coping strategies, (3) exploring coping resources, (4) teaching drink/target behavior refusal skills, and (5) setting the stage for the Relapse Prevention Phase of treatment. A variety of role-play techniques are introduced to help clients practice new coping skills. The Middle Treatment Phase concludes with a review of the therapy process, and an acknowledgment of successes and areas for improvement.

Chapter 7 outlines the Relapse Prevention Phase of treatment with the following goals: (1) evaluating clients' progress and assessing abstinence, (2) exploring clients' support network and providing recommendations for enhancement, (3) prioritizing recovery needs, and (4) creating individualized Action Plans to address recovery needs.

Chapter 8 contains various options on which to focus in the Relapse Prevention Phase. There are seven "Options" introduced in this chapter that clients may choose to work on in order to enhance their sobriety: Nutrition and Sobriety, Sexuality and Sobriety, Sleep and Sobriety, Work and Sobriety, Exercise and Sobriety, Smoking Cessation and Sobriety, and

Relaxation and Sobriety. Each of these topics includes a rationale, suggested procedures, and out-of-session exercises.

Chapter 9 outlines the End of Treatment Phase with the following goals: (1) discussing termination of treatment, (2) creating a long-term Recovery Plan, and (3) concluding therapy successfully.

Appendices and Forms are included at the end of the book. The appendices, in general, augment special topics introduced in the earlier chapters, and the forms are provided as tools for therapists to utilize during treatment.

CHAPTER 2

Special Considerations for Treating Alcoholic Women

Much of what we, as clinicians and researchers, know about alcoholism is based on studies of male alcoholics (Blume, 1986). Historically, women alcoholics have been underrepresented in research studies regardless of their increasing numbers in society (Vannicelli, 1984; Vannicelli & Nash, 1984). Lack of women's representation in research has led to a sketchy understanding of the special considerations of women with alcohol problems.

According to current statistics, fewer women than men drink. Estimates of the general population indicate that 15.1 million individuals are alcohol-abusing or alcohol-dependent. The number of women alcoholics or alcohol abusers ranges from 4.6 million to about 6 million (Roth, 1991), approximately one third of the population of alcoholics. The membership surveys conducted every 3 years by the General Services Office of AA reveal an increasing proportion of women reporting problems with alcohol. Although women still remain underrepresented in studies of members of AA (Beckman, 1993), percentages of women AA members indicate an increase: from 22% in 1968, to 30% in 1983, to 34% in 1986 (AA, 1987). This upsurge of alcoholism in women coincides with a steady rise in the number of women in treatment programs (Gomberg, 1981). In the areas of both research and treatment, there appears to be a gradual increase in the amount of attention given to women alcoholics (Dunne, 1988; Gomberg, 1987; Piazza, Vrbka, & Yeager, 1989; Roth, 1991; Schlesinger, Susman, & Koenigsberg, 1990; L.

14

Smith, 1992) and to women alcoholics in marital relationships (e.g., McCrady et al., 1986; B. A. Miller, 1990; B. A. Miller, Downs, & Gondoli, 1989; Noel, McCrady, Stout, & Fisher-Nelson, 1991). Although statistics indicate that alcoholic females marry as frequently as females in the general population (Perodeau, 1984), our understanding of married alcoholic women, and which treatment is best suited to this group, still remains incomplete and inadequate.

Over a decade ago, Wilsnack and colleagues (R. W. Wilsnack, Wilsnack, & Klassen, 1984) conducted the first full-scale survey on women's drinking patterns. Although the survey revealed no evidence of a general increase in alcohol consumption by women from 1960 to 1980, the survey did identify several subgroups of women with relatively high rates of drinking problems. Drinking behavior and problems associated with drinking are increased for women who are (1) unemployed and looking for work, (2) divorced or separated, (3) unmarried but living with a partner, (4) in their 20s and early 30s (also see Hilton, 1987), and (5) with heavy drinking husbands or partners. A woman's drinking behavior will, in general, parallel that of her husband, her siblings, or her close friends (R. W. Wilsnack et al., 1984).

There are a number of factors clinicians must be aware of when treating women alcoholics within the context of couple treatment. These factors fall into six central domains: (1) drinking and help-seeking behavior, (2) psychiatric history and current stressors, (3) physiological vulnerability to effects of alcohol, (4) reproductive complications, (5) marital/family functioning and parenting, (6) domestic violence, and (7) cultural factors in alcoholism.

DRINKING AND HELP-SEEKING BEHAVIOR

Women represent 25% of alcoholism clients in traditional treatment centers in the United States (National Institute on Drug Abuse, 1990), compared to men, who represent over 70%. Although it appears that female alcoholics comprise a small proportion of the overall treatment population, the proportion of female alcoholics to male alcoholics in treatment is similar to the proportion of all female alcoholics to male alcoholics.

According to a number of writers in the field, women start drinking, and begin the pattern of alcohol abuse, later than male alcoholics yet generally present for treatment at about the same age as men. Once women have begun heavy drinking, they experience a shorter interval between initiation of drinking and the development of alcohol-related problems (Piazza et al., 1989).

The context in which drinking occurs has been shown to differ for men and women. For instance, in the middle and upper classes women are more likely than men to drink alone and in the home (Blume, 1986; Schmidt, Klee, & Ames, 1990). Traditionally, these women have sought the help of their private physicians (rather than alcohol treatment programs) more so than have their male counterparts (Beckman & Kocel, 1982). As a result, alcoholic women are more frequently given mood-modifying drugs such as tranquilizers (e.g., Valium) than are male alcoholics. Consequently, by the time alcoholism is diagnosed, these women may have developed a cross-addiction to both alcohol and prescription drugs.

A variety of factors mitigate against women seeking alcohol treatment. Stigmatization of women's drinking leads to a tendency for women to drink alone and for them to be reluctant to identify as alcoholics. Furthermore, many alcoholic women are concerned that they may be be judged as incompetent mothers and/or lose their children, if they acknowledge that they have a serious drinking problem. Silence within families offers a false protection for female alcoholics.

Whereas men are generally encouraged to seek treatment by their wives, women historically have more often been encouraged to pursue treatment by their parents or children (Gomberg, 1974). Once a women has decided on treatment, one of the most frequently reported barriers she faces is lack of child care (S. C. Wilsnack, 1982). Finally, fewer women than men reach treatment through the court system or through employee assistance programs (Roman, 1988). All of these factors have adversely affected the number of women entering and remaining in alcoholism treatment programs.

The reasons that women enter treatment are more likely to be health, family, and/or relationship problems, whereas for men the reasons are more likely to be job and legal problems, especially Driving Under the Influence (DUI) or Driving While Intoxicated (DWI) (Lutz, 1991). Further, relative to their levels of alcohol/drug use, women are more likely than men to report psychological problems associated with alcohol/drug use; however, men are more likely to report problems of social functioning (Robbins, 1989).

In sum, clinicians must be aware that drinking and help-seeking behaviors differ for men and women and that these differences may have an impact on the point at which women initiate treatment, the reasons why women initiate treatment, and the concerns faced by women who have initiated treatment for alcoholism. Understanding the obstacles to the initiation of treatment faced by many alcoholic women is crucial for developing sensitive and effective treatment and long-term recovery planning.

PSYCHIATRIC HISTORY
AND CURRENT STRESSORS

Over the last decade, our awareness that individuals who are diagnosed with alcoholism often experience concomitant psychiatric disorders has increased (Hesselbrock & Hesselbrock, 1993; McCrady & Raytek, 1993). Psychological problems in alcohol-dependent individuals include, but are not limited to, depression, suicidal ideation and attempts, anxiety, posttraumatic stress (invariably the consequence of childhood sexual abuse or adult sexual assault), eating disorders, other drug abuse, as well as experiences of shame and guilt. *Depression* is one of the most frequently occurring symptoms associated with alcoholism (Hesselbrock & Hesselbrock, 1993; L. Smith, 1992), with prevalence rates ranging from 30–70% (Schuckit & Monteiro, 1988) in individuals who are alcohol-dependent. Women appear to experience depressive mood and ideation (Windle & Miller, 1989) and major depression (Hesselbrock, Meyer, & Keener, 1985) in greater numbers than their male counterparts. Some research indicates that depression precedes the development of alcoholism among women, especially those who are hospitalized (Hesselbrock et al., 1985; Schmidt et al., 1990), as compared to men. Other studies (e.g., Turnbull & Gomberg, 1988) assert that alcohol's depressant effect upon the central nervous system predisposes alcohol-dependent women to depressive disorders.

Closely associated with incidence of depression and alcoholism is the occurrence of *suicide attempts and suicides.* According to Hesselbrock, Hesselbrock, Syzmanski, and Weidenman (1988) suicide attempts were correlated with a lifetime diagnosis of major depressive disorder in both female and male (hospitalized) alcoholics; however, the prevalence of a lifetime diagnosis of major depression was higher among the women than the men in both suicide-attempt and nonattempt groups. In comparing alcoholic women under 40 years of age to their nonalcoholic counterparts, Gomberg (1989) found that the alcoholic women were almost five times more prone to suicide attempts.

Anxiety is a symptom experienced by many alcoholic women either before or after the onset of alcoholism. In a community sample of alcoholic women, the prevalence of a diagnosable panic or phobic disorder is two to three times more likely as compared to their nonalcoholic counterparts (Helzer & Pryzbeck, 1988). In a hospital sample of alcoholic women (Hesselbrock et al., 1985), as many as 44% of the women experience phobic disorders (such as agoraphobia; social, specific, and mixed phobias), and 14% of the women experienced panic disorders. It is important to note that psychiatric symptoms such as depression, anxiety, irritability, paranoia, and anger may be exacerbated between bouts of drinking

(Hesselbrock et al., 1985) as well as in the early phases of abstinence from alcohol.

Posttraumatic stress disorder, generally as a result of early childhood sexual abuse or more recent sexual assault, may also predispose women to abuse alcohol (Hurley, 1991; Rohsenow, Corbett, & Devine, 1988; S. C. Wilsnack, 1991; S.C. Wilsnack & R. W. Wilsnack, 1993) and other drugs. Estimates are that as many as 70% of women in treatment for alcohol and drug problems report histories of incest (Schaefer & Evans, 1987), rape, or other types of sexual abuse. A vicious cycle exists in which disturbing, and often debilitating, consequences of childhood sexual abuse—such as depression, low self-esteem, conflicted relationships, and sexual dysfunction—increase a woman's risk of self-medicative use of alcohol and other drugs (S. A. Russell & S. C. Wilsnack, 1991). The alcoholic woman is more likely than the alcoholic man to attribute the onset of pathological drinking to a particularly stressful life event. Events such as the loss of a pregnancy, the loss of a child due to illness or accident, the loss of a spouse or parent, a separation or divorce, or any dramatic, life-altering event can manifest as symptoms of posttraumatic stress and appear to be triggers for increased and out-of-control drinking. The inability to cope with these events may be exacerbated by a less than adequate support system and an inability to get and sustain psychological help. A focus on these issues, and on the subsequent constellation of posttraumatic stress symptoms, as risk factors for alcohol and other drug problems is key to successful prevention efforts for both young and adult women (Roth, 1991). In addition, a better understanding of those women who experience childhood sexual abuse (see Beutler, Williams, & Zetzer, 1994) or other dramatically stressful life events yet who do not manifest alcoholism or other drug addiction in adulthood would be a fruitful avenue of research in our expanding knowledge about the treatment and recovery needs of women.

It has been found that women who exhibit *eating-disordered behavior* may also experience pronounced drinking problems (see Krahn, 1993, for a review of studies of comorbidity of eating disorders and substance abuse). Although women with eating disorders use and abuse a variety of drugs, alcohol is the drug they most frequently abuse. Of the eating disorders, bulimia may well be the most researched and has been documented to have a strong relationship with alcoholism and other drug abuse. It is estimated that about one third of women receiving treatment for bulimia indicate a history of, or ongoing problem with, drug and alcohol abuse (Brisman & Siegel, 1984; Peveler & Fairburn, 1990). A smaller percentage of women with anorexia nervosa have substance abusing difficulties (e.g., Henzel, 1984). As a consequence to the prevalence of eating disorders in the population of women substance abusers, it is indicated that "eating behaviors should be assessed in all women presenting for any type of substance abuse" (Krahn, 1993, p. 296).

The *use and abuse of other psychoactive substances* has frequently been correlated with alcohol dependence in the general population and in women in particular. Women are twice as likely as men to use mood-altering prescription medications with alcohol, a potentially lethal combination (Roth, 1991). Additionally, alcoholic women are more likely to present with histories of other substance abuse, especially tranquilizers, sedatives, and amphetamines.

Another area in which gender differences occur in substance abuse is in the experience and outcome of *guilt and shame*. Women are more likely to deal with guilt and shame by internalizing their painful emotions. Whereas men act out their problems more directly (Gomberg, 1987), by getting into trouble with the law or by experiencing difficulty in social settings, women attempt to deal with internalized shame and guilt by self-medicating with alcohol and/or other drugs.

In summary, women alcoholics seem to constitute an identifiable group with a unique configuration of symptoms that may include low self-esteem, anxiety, depression, eating-disordered behavior, posttraumatic stress (possibly resulting from early or recent sexual abuse), other drug use, or shame and guilt. Treatment approaches need to establish therapeutic goals consistent with these symptoms and to design specific methods of addressing such symptoms (Schlesinger et al., 1990). A cognitive-behavioral approach to the treatment of alcoholism in women provides a direct way to address and manage symptoms such as those mentioned in this section by linking antecedent thoughts and feelings with drinking behavior. Helping women recognize when they use alcohol and other drugs as a way to cope with underlying symptoms is a first step in altering drinking behaviors and developing healthier means of coping with difficult psychological symptoms and current sequelae. In addition, treating women in the context of couple therapy may serve to enhance their support network.

PHYSIOLOGICAL VULNERABILITY TO THE EFFECTS OF ALCOHOL

Recent research on the impact of alcohol on women indicates that women's bodies are more biologically vulnerable to the effects of alcohol than are men's (Hill, 1984; Lieber, 1993; Roth, 1991). Some of the reasons thought to play a major role in women's biological vulnerability are life event stressors, poor nutrition, differences in metabolism, a pattern of more continuous drinking as compared to binge drinking, body weight or body water content, hormonal factors, genetic factors, the use of oral contraceptives, and the excessive use of over-the-counter drugs (Johnson, 1991).

An important early finding suggests that women reach higher peak levels of alcohol in the blood than men, even when they are given the same amount of absolute alcohol per pound of body weight (B. M. Jones & Jones, 1976). This occurs in part because women have a higher fat content and lower water content in their bodies than do men. Therefore, the alcohol consumed by women is dissolved in less total body water (Johnson, 1991).

Although women consume less alcohol on average than men, the effects of drinking can be devastating to women. Women alcoholics are more likely to suffer from anemia, circulatory disorders, and liver cirrhosis, and to commit suicide than alcoholic men. With respect to liver disease, women appear to develop more severe forms of liver disease than their male counterparts, and they are said to develop them more rapidly. Women appear to incur liver damage with shorter drinking histories and at lower levels of alcohol intake (even accounting for differences in body weight) than men (Johnson, 1991; see Lieber, 1993, for a review). It is important to note that there are both gender and ethnic group differences in the occurrence of liver disease and cirrhosis mortality rates: average age-adjusted death rates for chronic liver disease and cirrhosis from 1979–1981, for example (expressed as cases/100,000), were 6.9 for white females, 13.5 for black females, 15.4 for white males, and 29.4 for black males (Ronan, 1986–1987). Alcoholic women are more frequently disabled and for longer periods than alcoholic men. In addition, there is some evidence that drinking one ounce of absolute alcohol or more daily is associated with increased risk for breast cancer (Longnecker, Berlin, Orza, & Chalmers, 1988; Lowenfels & Zevola, 1989). Overall, women alcoholics have a higher death rate than their male peers (Hill, 1984).

Evidence from recent research indicates that alcohol consumption that may be considered "moderate and innocuous in men is not necessarily so in women" (Lieber, 1993, p. 11). Factors of physiological vulnerability are important to consider in assessing and treating women with drinking problems and may account for the higher incidence of somatic concerns experienced by women alcohol abusers. Clearly, an important component to assessment of alcoholic women is a comprehensive medical evaluation. An important component to cognitive-behavioral treatment is education on the biological vulnerability women must contend with in the consumption of alcohol.

REPRODUCTIVE COMPLICATIONS

There are a number of reproductive problems that women alcoholics and their offspring may experience in the span of the women's reproductive years. These difficulties include, but are not limited to, Fetal Alcohol Effects (FAE) and Fetal Alcohol Syndrome (FAS) in offspring, miscarriages, premature births, prenatal and postnatal complications, spontaneously induced abortions, stillbirths (S. C. Wilsnack, Klassen, & Wilsnack, 1984), and reduced fertility (Liepman et al., 1993).

Alcohol has been the most studied of all drugs during pregnancy (Geller, 1991b). The most dramatic effect of alcohol on the developing fetus is FAS, which is a cluster of birth defects resulting from the mother's abuse of alcohol during pregnancy. The diagnostic criteria for FAS include "growth deficiency, a characteristic pattern of physical malformations, central nervous system dysfunction, and mental retardation" (LaDue, 1991, p. 27). Studies have shown that FAS occurs at the rate of 1 in 759 births for the general population (Abel & Sokol, 1987). However, the incidence of FAS in some high-risk populations, such as Native Americans, may be as high as 1 in 50 births (May & Hymbaugh, 1983).

More pervasive than FAS are FAE, which are the less severe fetal problems resulting from woman's alcohol intake. These effects include "intrauterine growth retardation (the infants are small), smaller head circumference (microcephaly), increased anomalies, and, of great concern, impaired mental abilities" (Geller, 1991b, p. 102). Although FAE is less severe than FAS, children with this disorder suffer substantial developmental impairment throughout their lives. Thus, women who have been drinking alcohol during pregnancy also may have the additional challenge of parenting a child with moderate to severe developmental impairments. Although there is still controversy over how much drinking during pregnancy is innocuous, most researchers in the field caution that there is *no known safe level of alcohol consumption and no safe time during pregnancy in which to drink alcohol* (Little & Ervin, 1984). Exposure to fetal alcohol has been deemed "the most common preventable cause of mental retardation" (Taysi, 1988). Women who are alcohol-dependent may have confounding factors "such as lack of or inconsistent prenatal care, malnutrition, liver disease, infection, intoxication, withdrawal, trauma, and other drug exposure" (Liepman et al., 1993) that increase the risk for fetal complications.

A number of studies have indicated the relationship between alcohol and spontaneous abortions (see Little & Wendt, 1993, for a review). Risks of spontaneous abortion in the second trimester increase to twice as likely with the consumption of one to two drinks daily (Harlap & Shiono, 1980); some researchers have found that as few as one to two drinks weekly increases risk (Kline, Shrout, Stein, Susser, & Warburton, 1980).

For women alcoholics, the use of birth control also has its problems. Women who take oral contraceptives have been found to metabolize alcohol more slowly than women not using this form of birth control (M.

K. Jones & Jones, 1984). Therefore, women taking oral contraceptives experience the effects of alcohol to a greater degree and for a longer period of time than those who do not.

In sum, moderate or heavy alcohol use can have a significant impact on women's reproductive health and the health of their children throughout the lifespan. It is especially important to discuss with women the harmful consequences alcohol has during and beyond the reproductive years. Treatment for the woman and her partner that focuses on reproductive education and alternate behavior patterns will be beneficial for the health and well-being of the entire family unit.

MARITAL/FAMILY FUNCTIONING AND PARENTING

Experts agree that alcoholic women have more marital difficulties than do women in the general population (Perodeau, 1984). Alcoholic women are more likely to be divorced when they enter treatment or to be married to or living with an alcoholic "significant other." More often than alcoholic men, alcoholic women report marital difficulties as a cause for their drinking. It has not been ascertained, however, that marriages involving an alcoholic wife are necessarily more unstable than those involving an alcoholic husband (Perodeau, 1984). Both types of marriages appear to be unstable, although the instability may be expressed in different ways.

Partners of alcoholics are often heavy drinkers themselves. There is increasing evidence of a strong positive relationship between women's alcohol use and that of her partner or husband (e.g., Corbett, Mora, & Ames, 1991; Hammer & Vaglum, 1989; Jacob & Bremer, 1986). Research findings indicate women's frequency and amount of alcohol consumption is influenced by the alcohol consumption of their male partners (S. C. Wilsnack & Wilsnack, 1993) to a greater degree than men's alcohol consumption is influenced by the drinking behaviors of their female partners.

Noel and associates (1991) examined the marital functioning of alcoholics who seek outpatient therapy for alcohol and marital problems. Participants were assessed in terms of their marital and drinking histories, marital functioning, and marital satisfaction. Generally, male alcoholics were already drinking at the time of the marriage, whereas women alcoholics started drinking after the marriage and did not develop alcohol problems until later than their spouses did. Measures of marital functioning suggested that couples with an alcoholic wife were more satisfied with each other and themselves in their role functioning than were couples with an alcoholic husband. An observational measure of interaction revealed that alcoholic wives engaged in more positive communication with their husbands, whereas alcoholic husbands were more negative toward their wives.

Women who have a variety of different roles both within and outside the home tend to have lower incidence of alcohol problems than women who do not have multiple roles (S. C. Wilsnack, Wilsnack, & Klassen, 1986). Evidence suggests that role deprivation—that is, the loss of the role of worker, mother, or wife—may heighten a woman's risk for alcohol abuse (R. W. Wilsnack & Cheloha, 1987). Clinical experience also suggests that some women may experience certain roles, such as that of housewife or mother, as limiting and complain of a lack of purpose in life as a consequence. The experience of emptiness can be profound and may exacerbate drinking behavior as women try to diminish these painful thoughts and feelings.

Research on the effects of drinking on sexual responsiveness in women presents a striking paradox: actual alcohol consumption appears to decrease women's physiological sexual arousal while at the same time increasing their self-reported subjective sexual arousal. Wilsnack and colleagues (S. C. Wilsnack et al., 1984) suggests that it is important to study alcohol's disinhibiting effects on women's sexual cognitions and behaviors, including their feelings of subjective sexual arousal and their resulting sexual activity. For women these subjective cognitive effects may play a greater role in reinforcing and maintaining drinking behavior than do changes in objective physiological sexual arousal.

These findings have important implications for the treatment of alcoholic women seeking couple therapy. Interactions between the woman and her partner may mask underlying relationship dissatisfaction. Women partnered with heavy drinkers may be increasing their alcohol intake in an attempt to "keep up" with their partners' drinking behavior. Women who drink appear to be getting mixed messages in their bodies and minds with regard to sexual behavior. An important step in couple therapy would be to help women integrate their thoughts and feelings about their relationships, and to explore how their partners' drinking affects their own levels of alcohol consumption.

DOMESTIC VIOLENCE

Another critical issue for women is the devastating and potentially long-lasting effects of alcoholism on the family unit. For instance, alcohol and other drug problems contribute to at least 50% of spousal abuse, and up to 38% of child abuse (Roth, 1991). Recent studies indicate that women who are problem drinkers are more likely than nonalcoholic women to be the recipients of negative verbal interaction, as well as moderate or severe violence from a partner or spouse (B. A. Miller et al., 1989; O'Farrell & Murphy, 1995). Furthermore, women who are problem drinkers are more likely than their nonalcoholic peers to be the recipients of the alcohol-related sexual aggression of others (Blume, 1986; Frieze & Schaefer, 1984).

B. A. Miller (1990) presented research findings from studies that explored the relationships between family violence and alcohol or other drug problems. The following three forms of family violence were considered: child abuse, childhood sexual abuse, and spousal violence. These findings indicated that (1) women alcoholics were more likely than the general population of women to be the recipients of spousal violence, (2) alcohol problems in women contributed to the frequency and severity of spousal violence these women experienced, (3) alcohol problems in parents were related to abuse of their children, and (4) childhood sexual abuse was related to the later development of alcohol problems in women (B. A. MIller, 1990).

When assessing and treating alcoholic women in a marital or relationship context, it is critical to inquire about the occurrence of domestic violence, both past and present, including the frequency and severity of any abuse. The beginning phases of treatment should always clarify with both women and their partners that violence in the home is unacceptable. Interventions should focus on ways to alter violent behavior, such as leaving the setting, meeting up later to discuss the problem, or waiting to discuss the problem with the therapist.

CULTURAL FACTORS IN ALCOHOLISM

It is clear from the literature that women have been tragically underserved, both in prevention and in treatment programs; women of color have been especially disregarded (Roth, 1991). The following cultural factors are especially important for further understanding and treating alcoholism in women.

The fastest growing minority group in the United States is individuals of Hispanic background, who currently constitute about 9% of the U.S. population (Liepman et al., 1993). Because Hispanic culture represents diverse groups of people, it is difficult to generalize results of studies of one group to that of another. Generally speaking, patterns of substance abuse of foreign-born Hispanics parallel those of their homeland compatriots, whereas substance abuse patterns of Hispanics born in the United States look more like those of the dominant culture (Cervantes, Gilbert, de Snyder, & Padilla, 1991). In Latin American women, variations in alcohol use are associated with generational status, age, acculturation (Mora & Gilbert, 1991), education, marital status, income, and birthplace (Caetano, 1986–1987, 1990; Caetano & Mora, 1988). Latinas who are born in the United States, who are acculturated into Western culture, who have achieved above average socioeconomic status, and who are middle aged tend to have increased drinking behavior patterns (Caetano, 1990; Holck, Warren, Smith, & Rochat, 1984), whereas women who are less acculturated tend more frequently to be abstainers.

Studies on the patterns of substance use and abuse in African American women have been disconcertingly scarce. Information that is available tends to focus on women in high-density, low socioeconomic vicinities and tends to have small sample sizes making it difficult to generalize findings to African American women in other settings (Herd, 1989). According to recent survey findings, African American women are more inclined to abstain from alcohol (e.g., M. Russell, 1989) than Caucasian women. However, in the subset of African American women who do drink, they tend to drink heavily and to sustain more alcohol-related difficulties (Caetano, 1984). African American women who have a heavy pattern of drinking tend to be older (45–59 years old) as contrasted to Caucasian women (25–44 years old) (Lillie-Blanton, Mackenzie, & Anthony, 1991; M. Russell, 1989), tend to be unemployed and looking for work (M. Russell, 1989), and tend to have a household income of less than $6,000 per year (Lillie-Blanton et al., 1991). With respect to education, unlike Hispanic American women, African American women who have a college degree or beyond are less likely than their Caucasian counterparts to exhibit heavy drinking patterns (Liepman et al., 1993). For African American women, the issues that place this group at risk for problems with alcohol and drugs are precisely the issues that affect their ability to seek help. The African American woman receives very little prevention information and treatment, yet is most frequently punished for behavior accompanying alcohol and other drug abuse (such as drinking during pregnancy) (Taha-Cisse, 1991). Liepman et al. (1993) recommend that once African American women enter treatment, mental health care providers address their "survival needs including employment, health, safety, clothing, housing, legal and school-related issues" (p. 222). Central to the treatment of the African American female client is an assessment of her partner's drinking behavior, and her involvement in nuclear and extended family networks (Liepman et al., 1993) and religious organizations. There is evidence to suggest that directive, cognitive, and action oriented treatment approaches are the most useful for this group of alcohol abusers (Harper, 1984).

Alcohol abuse and its consequences are perhaps the most destructive force affecting the health and well-being of Native Americans (Liepman et al., 1993). Native Americans are quite diverse, although they represent less than 1% of the population of the United States, there are over 280 different cultural groups. Comprehensive statistics of drinking patterns vary considerably from "group to group, between urban areas, federal reservations, and isolated northern villages, and between men and women" (Liepman et al., 1993, p. 227). Native Americans suffer greater mortality rates due to alcoholism, and alcohol-related motor vehicle accidents, suicide, homicide, and cirrhosis of the liver than the general U.S. population (Liepman et al., 1993). Although Native American women drink less alcohol than their male counterparts, their deaths account for almost half of the deaths due to cirrhosis (Liepman et al., 1993). Native American women appear to be at a higher risk for alcohol abuse if they are away from their traditional centers of familial, spiritual, and communal support (LaDue, 1991), and if they are younger (Lemert, 1982). The loss of cultural ties and values contributes greatly to alcoholism in this group (LaDue, 1991). The triad of alcoholism, violence, and depression has been cited as the most serious social and health problem facing Native American women and their families today (LaDue, 1991).

Asian American women appear to be the least studied (Chi, Lubben, & Kitano, 1989), of the cultural groups presented in this section. This fact, coupled with the fact that Asian Americans are quite diverse (inclusive of individuals of Chinese, Japanese, Korean, and various other descents), makes our knowledge of the drinking behaviors of Asian American women incomplete. A review of national health surveys (S. C. Wilsnack & Wilsnack, 1993) indicated that Asian American women were the least likely of all ethnic subgroups (Caucasian, African American, Hispanic, and Native American) to be drinkers. However, because of the small sample sizes of the studies reviewed, caution should be taken in interpreting these, and many other, findings on the drinking patterns of culturally diverse women.

With respect to treatment, it is recommended that interventions be culturally competent, developed to meet the specific values of the woman, her extended family, and the community in which she lives (Liepman et al., 1993).

TREATMENT CONSIDERATIONS

Women with alcohol problems differ from their male counterparts in a number of important ways. Understanding the factors of (1) drinking and help-seeking behavior, (2) psychiatric history and current stressors, (3) physiological vulnerability to the effects of alcohol, (4) reproductive complications, (5) marital/family functioning and parenting, (6) domestic violence, and (7) the racial and ethnic diversity of women alcoholics will provide a framework for more effective prevention, intervention, and treatment services. Women with alcohol problems need comprehensive treatment services that take into consideration the complexity of alcohol-'ism as well as the medical, psychological, economic, and cultural needs of women, their partners, and their children. It is likely that an alcoholic women will not begin or continue treatment in a program that misunderstands or fails to recognize significant facets of her life (McCrady & Raytek, 1993).

Although our knowledge of the special treatment needs of women with alcohol problems is increasing (see McCrady & Raytek, 1993, for a review), there is still a scarcity of research on women compared to that on men. For instance, women with drinking problems continue to represent only a minority of treatment outcome research (McCrady & Raytek, 1993; Vannicelli, 1984).

Due to the many demands placed on women within the family, within the work environment, and within the community, outpatient rather than inpatient treatment programs appear to be the most practical for many women with alcohol problems (Roth, 1991), unless the woman is suicidal or in need of detoxification, in which cases, inpatient services are indicated. It is easier to find part-time than full-time child care and less disruptive for the woman and her family when she decides to seek outpatient services. It is also less economically disruptive, because women can often continue working during treatment and because hospital inpatient programs are more expensive. These points are inherent in the intensive program outlined in this manual, which makes this 20-session outpatient model an ideal treatment for alcoholic women in relationships.

ACUTE PHASE

CHAPTER 3

Phase I: Preparation for Treatment

Overview

Rapport Building
Confidentiality
Substance Use History
Substance Abuse Treatment and Psychiatric Treatment History
Treatment Expectations
Confirmation of Abstinence and the Behavioral Contract

Materials Needed:

- ◆ Behavioral Contracts
- ◆ Pencils and Clipboards
- ◆ Business Card with Emergency Phone Numbers

Recommended number of sessions: 3

Goals: *1. Build rapport with clients.*
        2. Establish confidentiality parameters.
        3. Gather relevant history.
        4. Prepare clients for therapy.
        5. Come to agreement on therapeutic goals, and create Behavioral Contracts.
        6. Decide on time and frequency of sessions.

In the initial sessions with clients, the following issues should be attended to: (1) rapport building with clients, (2) issues of confidentiality, (3) exploration of past and present alcohol and other drug use by both partners, (4) exploration of past treatment attempts, (5) exploration of treatment expectations, and (6) agreement regarding therapeutic goals. In addition, deciding on the time and frequency of sessions is important.

Appendix 1 offers a suggested meeting schedule if the therapist chooses to follow the 20-session model recommended in this book. The recommended meeting schedule was developed to provide intense treatment in the Early Treatment Phase, and moves to a less frequent meeting schedule during the Middle Treatment Phase. As therapy continues into the Relapse Prevention Phase and End of Treatment Phase, sessions begin to taper off, allowing for the integration of skills into the clients' daily lives. The Relapse Prevention Phase is particularly designed to allow clients plenty of time to bring difficulties back to treatment in order to work them through, as well as time to reinforce successes.

RAPPORT BUILDING
The Alcoholic Client

A good rapport with the client is, of course, necessary before session goals can be accomplished. Building rapport with alcoholic clients and partners of alcoholics can bring about a few challenges worth mentioning. The first issue to be aware of with the alcoholic client is the origin of his or her motivation at the beginning of treatment. Often, the first treatment episode for an alcoholic is triggered by a crisis—marital or legal, job- or health-related. Thus, the alcoholic's motivation for abstinence and participation in therapy may simply be to end the crisis, resolve the immediate problem(s), and alleviate the emotional pain. If this is the case, the alcoholic will often want to accomplish these goals and continue to drink, albeit drink less and with more control. It may take a few weeks, months, and in some cases, a few treatment episodes before the alcoholic realizes that this goal is futile. This realization, or "surrender," as it is referred to in recovery programs, is the point at which a deeper level of motivation and commitment to change can really begin. Uncovering the motivation level and true goals of the client is an important focus of the first few treatment sessions.

Thus, if an alcoholic client enters treatment with this tenuous motivation and lack of commitment to abstinence, his or her attitude is likely to be wary and defensive. This will be especially true when the partner or the legal system "recommended" the treatment. Building rapport under these conditions is often difficult. Frequently, the alcoholic will question the therapist regarding his or her credentials and training. In particular, the alcoholic client will often want to know whether or not the therapist is a recovering alcoholic. Regardless of the way in which the client expresses his or her defensiveness and wariness, it is important to understand the underlying fears the client is attempting to ease. Common concerns the alcoholic client has in the beginning stages of treatment are fears of being judged and stereotyped, fears of detoxification, fears of being "forced" to quit drinking with no other way to deal with problems, and shame regarding past behavior. The client may also be concerned about his or her relationship and having to face the partner's anger, pain, and resentment. Thus, it is important to explore these concerns with clients as they surface, directly or indirectly, and let clients know that these issues will be addressed in therapy.

The foregoing description of the defensive client usually holds true when this is his or her first treatment episode and/or the client has been coerced, threatened, or required to attend therapy. However, clients who have had numerous treatment episodes, and/or enter therapy of their own accord, present a different challenge. In this case, the clients may have an attitude of hopelessness, helplessness, and shame. They have "surrendered" to the fact that they cannot continue to drink, but are at a loss as to how to maintain abstinence. Building rapport with this type of client involves empathizing with his or her discouragement, while at the same time letting the client know that there is hope. Many alcoholics struggle with maintaining abstinence because they have not learned to identify high-risk situations, and have not learned the necessary coping skills to deal with these difficult situations. Having the client understand this is important in helping him or her move beyond initial feelings of helplessness. This approach also helps to lessen the shame that clients may be experiencing and can give them a sense of control in the recovery process; that is, instilling in them the idea that there is indeed something they can "do" to help themselves. Furthermore, being in couple therapy is highly advantageous for the client because there is strong evidence of the effectiveness of this approach for the treatment of alcoholism (McCrady et al., 1986; O'Farrell, 1991).

The Partner

Working with the alcoholic's defensiveness and resistance to treatment and building rapport with him or her will be an ongoing concern, but it is essential to address it in the first session before moving forward. In addition, building rapport with the partner is also critical and may raise a different set of obstacles. On the one hand, the partner may be in collusion with the alcoholic and present a wary, defensive stance, denying the extent of the problem and looking for a "quick fix." On the other hand, the partner may be relieved finally to have some help in addressing the alcohol problem, but may also be resistant to looking at his or her own contributions to the problem. Another common scenario is one in which the partner presents with a great deal of anger and resentment with little motivation to participate in the treatment. Regardless of the presentation, it is critical to address the parent's concerns, reflect the feelings being expressed, and attempt to normalize the reactions of the couple to entering treatment.

The Couple

Offering therapy to a couple, when one partner is alcoholic, can be a setup for the alcoholic to play out the role of the "identified patient." When this happens, there is often a tug-of-war between clients for the therapist's alliance. (Note: This can also occur when both partners are in treatment for alcoholism and one partner's condition is more severe.) Thus, identifying this behavior pattern and intervening immediately is critical for the couple's therapy to progress and the goals to be achieved. Although it is important to maintain the focus of helping the alcoholic abstain from alcohol and other drugs, it is just as important to help the partner identify those behaviors she or he has developed that reinforce a drinking lifestyle. The partner needs to be an active participant in every session; indeed, the purpose of the "target behavior" is to allow the partner to engage in a parallel process with the alcoholic (see Chapter 1, p. 7). The therapist may need to continually reframe the alcoholism as a "couple issue" and point out how each partner contributes to the drinking lifestyle; that is, how each partner's verbal and nonverbal behavior either reinforces drinking or reinforces abstinence.

While helping the partner become aware of his or her role in the drinking behavior, it is imperative that this intervention is not interpreted to mean he or she *caused* the drinking. Many partners of alcoholics believe that they caused the alcoholism and readily accept blame from the alcoholic. In this case, the therapist can use this as an opportunity to point out that each partner needs to take responsibility for his or her own behavior in the relationship, and not for the alcoholism; blaming each other is not productive and prohibits a healthy, working relationship.

Note. When exploring client's motivations for treatment, it may become clear that the couple has significant marital/couple issues. If this is the case, we suggest that the therapist and clients agree on how these problems will be addressed early on in treatment so that treatment focus is maintained. The therapist can briefly cover the limitations of therapy given the focus on alcoholism treatment and explain to the couple that marital/couple issues will be addressed in the context of how they may affect drinking or engagement in the target behavior. It will be important, however, to assure the couple that any marital/couple issues that surface along the way can be set aside and discussed near the end of treatment. This allows a clear focus on the alcoholism. If the therapist has the competency to deal with such issues, he or she may choose to continue helping the couple work on their relationship. Another option, of course, is to give clients appropriate referrals for dealing with these lingering relationship issues. The main focus of the treatment approach outlined in this book is the cessation of drinking and a target behavior. Chapter 5 introduces a number of communication skills designed to enhance the couple's relationship and reinforce abstinence behavior. These skills may be very useful in addressing additional marital/couple concerns.

Case Illustration: Rapport Building

Background

Mike, a 42-year-old Caucasian male, and Beth, a 45-year-old Caucasian female, have been married for 5 years. It is the second marriage for each of them. Beth has two teenage boys, aged 14 and 16, from a previous marriage, living in the home. Mike works as an engineer at a local company; Beth works full time as a nurse in a nearby hospital. Mike has been drinking since he was 15 years old. His drinking became problematic during his early 30s which resulted in two DUIs and the end of his first marriage. He was able to cut down on his alcohol use for the next few years during which time he started a new job and began dating Beth.

Presenting Problem

At the time of the initial interview, the couple report Mike's drinking to have increased over the last 3 years in response to family problems and job stress. Beth is particularly distressed about Mike's increased drinking because she reports that her first husband was an abusive alcoholic. They have both agreed that Mike's abstinence from alcohol is the primary goal of treatment. However, they have chosen couple therapy to address this problem because they both acknowledge how much their relationship has been affected by Mike's drinking. Additionally, Mike and Beth recognize that there may be problems in their relationship that contribute to Mike's desire to drink and would like to work on their relationship through couple therapy.

It is clear in the first session that Beth has initiated the couple's entering treatment for Mike's alcohol problem. She attempts to get the therapist to validate her views on the destructiveness of Mike's drinking. If Mike would just stop drinking, Beth asserts, all of the family's problems would be resolved. Although Mike agrees with Beth that his drinking has increased, he is quick to point out that there are many problems in the family that have little to do with his drinking. Mike minimizes his drinking and attempts to get the therapist to focus on other family problems.

At this point, the therapist must explore what each partner's stated motivation is for treatment, as well as any underlying agendas. As the session progresses, the therapist becomes clear that Beth wants therapy to "fix Mike" and fantasizes that the relationship will be "perfect" once her husband stops drinking. While exploring Mike's motivation for treatment, the therapist uncovers that Mike wants his wife "off his back" and he believes that agreeing to therapy and abstinence will give him some relief from her constant criticism. It appears that in the long run Mike intends to control his drinking rather than become abstinent.

In order to build rapport with Beth, the therapist must begin to empathize with her fear of repeating her first marriage, to understand the impact Mike's drinking may have on her two sons, and to reinforce her desire to resolve the current stressors in their family life. In building rapport with Mike, the therapist must begin to empathize with Mike's anger that all of the family problems have been blamed on his drinking, to understand how he perceives his conflicts at work and home, and to reinforce his developing awareness that drinking may exacerbate his problems. In building rapport with the couple, the therapist must help Beth and Mike reframe the alcoholism and other family problems as couples' issues rather than as individual issues. In viewing the problems from a couple perspective both partners will be able to explore the behaviors that contribute to drinking and other difficulties in the relationship (e.g., poor communication). In addition, working together as a couple will provide a framework for exploring new behaviors that are supportive of abstinence and healthy relating.

CONFIDENTIALITY

When working with alcoholic couples, confidentiality issues can become tricky if they are not clearly addressed at the beginning of treatment and consistently enforced as therapy progresses. Families with alcoholics in them often hold secrets from each other, and one or both of the partners often attempt to include the therapist in the secret-holding. Thus, it is critical that agreements be made regarding confidentiality at the beginning of therapy and, if necessary, written into the Behavioral Contract (see Figures 3.1 and 3.2). Agreements regarding whether the therapist will see clients individually if there is a crisis or if one partner does not show up for the couple session should also be addressed. We suggest an "open" policy where *any* information may be shared with both clients if determined by the therapist to be important to treatment. This policy helps to reinforce a communication pattern that is conducive to sobriety in contrast to the secretive, manipulative pattern that is pervasive in active alcoholic families.

SUBSTANCE USE HISTORY

It is important to get a detailed history of substance use *from both partners.* One partner may be presenting with the alcohol problem, but the other may also have problems with alcohol or other substances. Obtaining this information can occur in individual sessions with each client or in a couple session. On the one hand, individual sessions with each partner may yield more accurate information regarding the amount and frequency of chemical use if the individual has a history of hiding his or her drinking or other drug use. On the other hand, having the partner present when giving information about substance use may yield more accurate information. This would be the case if the alcoholic is minimizing his or her drinking and the partner is able to provide a more realistic account of the drinking and/or other drug use. (In the former case where clients are seen individually for history taking, it is essential that the issue of confidentiality be addressed prior to obtaining a history.) We suggest the therapist ask about *all* illicit drug use and prescription medications, in addition to the alcohol use. When clients report having "tried" a particular substance or "occasionally" using a drug, it is important to determine what this means. If a client is having difficulty being specific, the therapist can always ask a question such as, "You said you occasionally use marijuana, does that mean a few times a week?" A good rule of thumb is to guess higher or more frequent use than likely to be the case. Alcoholic clients invariably underreport alcohol and other drug use at the beginning of treatment. It is not uncommon to discover other drug use or more extensive alcohol use after therapy has been in progress for a few weeks or months.

A detailed substance use history should include the following:

1. Type of drug(s) used (licit and illicit)—make sure to ask specifically about prescribed medications
2. Amount of drug(s) used
3. Frequency of drug use (both past and present)
4. Reaction to drug(s) (e.g., did client become intoxicated, hallucinate, become paranoid, etc.)
5. Withdrawal symptoms when drug use ceased

If clients are still using alcohol and/or other drugs, and have agreed to stop such use, it is critical to explore past experiences when they attempted to quit. *Detoxification from alcohol and other substances can be life threat-ening. A general guideline is to refer clients to a physician to monitor detoxification.*

SUBSTANCE ABUSE TREATMENT
AND PSYCHIATRIC TREATMENT HISTORY

After determining what substances have been used in the past and are currently used by both partners, the therapist can explore treatment approaches clients have previously attempted. Has the alcoholic been in a residential or inpatient program, intensive outpatient treatment, or psychotherapy in the past? Has the alcoholic sought treatment for any other psychological problems? How about the partner? Have they tried 12-step programs? All of this information is important to understanding the clients more fully. An alcoholic client seeking treatment for the first time may be very different from the alcoholic client who has been through numerous treatment programs in the past. Exploring the following areas can be very helpful in the therapist's treatment planning:

1. What approaches were the most and least helpful in the past?
2. How much sobriety was the client able to attain after treatment(s) and how did he or she maintain sobriety?
3. What is the client's understanding of relapse and is he or she able to identify triggers to drinking?
4. Has the partner participated with the alcoholic in past treatment?
5. Has either client been involved in psychiatric treatment of any kind, including seeing a psychologist; psychiatrist; marriage, family, and child counselor; or social worker?

As mentioned previously, clients who have sought treatment in the past and returned to drinking may present with a sense of hopelessness or disbelief that they can succeed at any treatment. Thus, it is important for the therapist to spend time gathering information, building rapport, and passing on a sense of hope to the clients.

Note. It is also important to obtain more general information that may be helpful in the current treatment. This information may include, but is not limited to, a history of the couple's relationship: the length of time married or in the relationship together and the quality of the relationship; history of domestic violence; history of previous significant relationships; history of family alcoholism and psychiatric illnesses; history of child abuse or exposure to traumatic events; legal problems related to alcohol or other drug use; psychosocial functioning; employment problems; and significant current or past health concerns.

TREATMENT EXPECTATIONS

Once the background information has been gathered regarding the presenting problem, substance use history, and past treatment attempts, the therapist should explore the clients' current treatment expectations and share his or her expectations for moving the therapy forward.

Client Expectations

With alcoholic couples, for whom secrets are common and indirect communication is often the norm, covert agendas are also to be expected. It is not unusual for the couple and/or one of the partners to have a hidden agenda for entering therapy. As mentioned in the earlier section on Building Rapport, the alcoholic client may have an agenda that involves learning how to drink "less," or with "more control" versus quitting drinking. Or, as is often the case when couples present for therapy, the alcoholic's agenda may be to appease his or her partner, at least temporarily, especially if the partner is threatening divorce. The partner may have an agenda for the therapist to "fix" the alcoholic; that is, to get him or her to quit drinking and solve the myriad problems that have developed over the years. The partner may or may not expect to be an active participant in therapy. Often one extreme or the other is presented where the partner either sees the alcoholic's drinking as the sole source of the problem, or sees his or her own behavior as the primary source of the problem.

Another possible difficulty occurs when the couple collude with each other and present an overt set of treatment expectations that involve abstinence and active participation in therapy, but continue to minimize the drinking and to emphasize other marital/couple issues. Thus, trying to uncover both the overt and covert agendas that the clients bring to therapy will be important in order to proceed successfully. While exploring the clients' expectations, we recommend covering the following issues:

1. How does the couple and each partner *benefit* from the alcoholic's drinking?
2. What are the *costs* to each partner and to the couple as a result of the drinking?
3. What does each partner and the couple have to *lose* if the alcoholic continues to drink?

4. What does each partner and the couple have to *gain* if the
   alcoholic quits drinking and maintains abstinence?

Case Illustration: Client Expectations

Beth and Mike have a difficult time, at first, answering the therapist's question
regarding how each of them *benefits* from Mike's drinking. Both partners
have been focused on the negative aspects of Mike's drinking for so long that
they are at a loss for what they may have *gained* by Mike's drinking.
Eventually, the couple are able to identify the following gains from Mike's
drinking: (1) They do not have to look at other aspects of their relationship
that are not working (e.g., poor communication, dissatisfying sexual relationship), which exist even when Mike was abstinent from alcohol; (2) Mike
is actually more affectionate with Beth and the children when he is drinking;
(3) Beth has someone to care for and focus on, which is important now that
her sons are older and more independent; and, (4) Mike is able to express his
emotions more readily when he is drinking, which is a difficult task for him
when abstinent from alcohol.

With relative ease, the couple is able to identify the *costs* to their
relationship, as well as to themselves individually, as a result of Mike's
drinking. Mike admits that although he feels more comfortable expressing
his emotions while drinking, he often goes overboard and becomes even more
uncomfortable. Additionally, Mike states that he occasionally blacks out and
forgets what he has said to his wife or to the children. Beth admits that
although it makes her feel good to take care of Mike, she also feels resentful
and feels that her needs are not being met. Both partners realize that the
communication and sexual problems they have are only made worse by the
alcohol.

Prior to coming in to treatment, Beth told Mike that if he did not seek
help, she would leave. She maintains this stance in therapy and firmly states
that if he drops out of treatment or continues to drink, she will leave. Mike
realizes that his relationship with Beth and her sons will be lost if he continues
to drink. He also realizes that he might lose his job and get into more legal
trouble if he continues to drink. It is during this conversation that Mike begins
to realize that his original motive of trying to control his drinking may be
futile.

Completing treatment and maintaining a sober lifestyle, Mike acknowledges, would keep his family intact, save his job, and keep him out of legal
trouble. He also states that he is "tired" of the hangovers, blackouts, and
regrets about his behavior. Quitting drinking for Mike "just might be a
relief." Beth is convinced that she would gain a better relationship with her
husband by participating in treatment. The therapist has to help Beth realize

that it is not her job to "fix" Mike and that they both have to work on this problem together. Additionally, the therapist has to help Beth see that quitting drinking will not "solve" all of their problems, that the couple has some work to do on their relationship in addition to Mike quitting drinking.

Helping the couple frame Mike's alcoholism as a "couple's issue" is helpful for both partners. Mike feels some relief that it is not only his problem and that Beth will have to take some responsibility for making changes herself. Beth feels pleased that there is a positive way to help Mike without enabling him to continue to drink.

Therapist Expectations

Each therapist will have his or her own expectations for therapy. We have included four general expectations for the therapy approach described in this book. The *first expectation* is that the alcoholism will be treated from a cognitive-behavioral perspective. The *second expectation* is that the alcoholic will be treated in the context of a couple and that both partners will learn how to support one another actively. The *third expectation* is that the alcoholic will abstain from alcohol and other drugs. The *fourth expectation* is that the partner will choose a behavior from which he or she will abstain (or decrease, if appropriate) throughout the program. We refer to the behavior from which the partner is abstaining as the "target behavior." The following section describes the rationale and the suggested procedures for introducing these expectations to clients.

Cognitive-Behavioral Approach to Alcoholism

The therapist can explain to clients that from the cognitive-behavioral perspective, drinking is a maladaptive behavior that has been reinforced over time. In reinforcing drinking behavior, alcoholics become less efficient in utilizing other coping skills when problems surface. Consequently, the alcoholic needs to learn more effective coping skills. This therapy approach teaches cognitive and behavioral strategies to help the alcoholic stop drinking, maintain abstinence, and improve the quality of his or her life. Furthermore, the program described in this manual works from the premise that the most effective approach is a collaborative one, whereby the clients and the therapist all take an active role in every session. Clients are routinely assigned out-of-session exercises to aid in the generalization of the learned skills from therapy to daily living. The clients are also taught how to set realistic goals for themselves and how to follow up on these goals to maximize their successes. Lastly, we emphasize the need for a "Recovery Plan," which that the clients create with the therapist toward the end of the program to reinforce new behaviors and increase the likelihood of continued abstinence.

Treatment in a Couple Context

The rationale for treating the alcoholic in the context of a couple is explained in detail in Chapter 1 and may be shared with the clients.

Abstinence from Alcohol

The rationale for having alcoholics choose abstinence as a treatment goal is explained in detail in Chapter 1 and may be shared with the clients. It is recommended that this expectation be explicit and that any resistance from the client or partner be explored as soon as possible.

Choosing a Target Behavior

The purpose of the partner decreasing or eliminating a behavior is twofold. First, research has shown that problem drinkers are more successful in increasing the number of days of abstinence and maintaining this gain when their partners are involved in treatment (McCrady et al., 1986). Second, it is our philosophy by participating in a parallel process to that of the alcoholic, the partner will develop more empathy and understanding for the alcoholic. Moreover, as the partner concentrates on decreasing or eliminating a behavior, then his or her energy will be positively redirected to a personal goal, rather than to the alcoholic's goal. For many partners, this self-focus is a challenge in and of itself, because they have learned over the years to direct a great deal of their attention toward the alcoholic. Because of the difficulty partners may have with focusing on themselves, they may have a hard time deciding on a target behavior. The following guidelines are offered to the therapist in order to help the partner choose an appropriate behavior from which to abstain (or to decrease).

1. On the one hand, partners may initially be resistant to choosing a target behavior because they are in treatment "for the alcoholic," not for themselves. If this is the case, this is a good opportunity to state the program rationale clearly and to reiterate the purpose of having the partner choose a target behavior. On the other hand, some partners are relieved to have a "purpose" in treatment and to focus on themselves "for a change." Take time to ensure that the target behavior is meaningful to the partner and that successful reduction or abstinence will yield increased self-esteem and confidence.

2. The chosen behavior is one that he or she will either *reduce* or *eliminate*. Examples include abstaining from coffee, sugar, soda, nicotine, or gambling/betting; or reducing sugar intake, TV time, or spending money.

3. The behavior must be *specific and concrete*. For example, if the partner wants to eliminate "overeating," help him or her to identify exactly what food is being consumed excessively or if he or she is eating too frequently (e.g., eating two bags of potato chips at work every day or eating snacks in the middle of the day). It is usually best to have the partner initially choose just one behavior from which to abstain, like eating snacks *or* eating desserts. If he or she is successfully able to maintain this abstinence, then choose another behavior. It is important to maximize the opportunity for success by beginning slowly.

4. The behavior must be *operationalized*; that is, the partner must have a clear picture of what it will look like when he or she is successful. For example, if the partner chooses "decreasing procrastination," it is very difficult to determine when she is successful and when she is not. Thus, a better way to frame this goal would be to reduce the amount of time she spends on "breaks" in her work schedule. With this goal, first help her figure out what her current average breaktime is, and then help her choose an appropriate amount of time for breaks. She would then work towards reducing the current breaktime to meet her goal.

5. The partner needs to choose a behavior that is *meaningful* to him or her and that is *separate from the alcoholic*. Some clients may want to eliminate "codependency" or "enabling." Let them know that there will be opportunity to work on these concerns in the program. For the target behavior, the partner must choose something that is independent of the alcoholic's drinking. The behavior chosen, however, may be affected by the alcoholic's drinking. For example, the partner may overeat when his wife begins drinking as a means of coping with stress. Clearly, his behavior is affected by the wife's drinking, but is most also likely triggered by other stressors and, thus, not completely focused on the alcoholic.

6. In helping the partner choose an appropriate target behavior, it may become clear that he or she has a clinically significant problem that needs addressing. For example, if a partner chooses "overeating" as a target behavior and then reveals that she binges and purges, further assessment of an eating disorder is indicated. If the therapist is the competent to treat such a problem, it may be incorporated into treatment, as long as the focus on the alcoholism is maintained. Otherwise, a referral may be in order.

7. Another possibility that may arise when the partner is choosing a target behavior is that he or she chooses to abstain from alcohol (or another drug) because he or she also has a drinking problem. If this is the

case, although there are a couple of important points to keep in mind. First, the client who presents as the "alcoholic" may have the more severe drinking problem, the couple may be minimizing the partner's drinking. Or the partner's drinking may be as serious a problem and deserve equal attention. The therapy approach outlined in this book is still appropriate, but both members' drinking problems should be addressed equally. A second point of concern is when both clients are in treatment for alcoholism and one partner continues to drink or relapses. The individual having difficulty maintaining abstinence may need to be referred to a more intensive treatment setting; in that case, treating both partners in couple therapy would be contraindicated.

CONFIRMATION OF ABSTINENCE AND THE BEHAVIORAL CONTRACT

During the Preparation Phase of treatment, it is very important to discuss the therapeutic goal of abstinence from alcohol and other drugs, as well as abstinence from, or reduction of, the partner's target behavior. In addition, formally contracting with clients to abstain from alcohol and other drugs can be an effective intervention. The following section describes the rationale for using a Behavioral Contract and the procedures for implementing this as a tool in the therapy program. Sample Behavioral Contracts are presented in Figures 3.1 and 3.2.

Rationale

The purpose of using a Behavioral Contract with clients is to enhance compliance with the treatment conditions and goals. The use of contracts between therapist and clients is a common strategy in the managing many client problems (Bongar, 1992; O'Farrell & Bayog, 1986). In addition to clarifying expectations and goals, a Behavioral Contract may be helpful to fall back on when a client is having difficulty adhering to the agreed-upon treatment. Writing the contract together may also serve to enhance the collaborative nature of the therapy and the likelihood that the contract is followed.

Procedure

Two types of contracts need to be considered: informed consent for therapy and Behavioral Contracts. Clients, of course, have the right to decide whether or not to enter psychotherapy and whether or not to continue in treatment. In order to make an intelligent decision, clients must understand the nature, costs, and benefits of treatment; the likelihood of success; and alternative methods of treatment. It is the ethical responsibility of the therapist to provide potential clients with this information. Increasingly, therapists are using written contracts to provide clients with information about therapy, about the limits of confidentiality, and about their freedom to withdraw from treatment at any time. These contracts are signed by the therapist and both clients. Alternatively, this information can be provided at the beginning of the first session. In either case, treatment and the responsibilities therein must be discussed in sufficient detail with the clients, and any questions should be answered prior to committing to treatment.

Because the purpose of the Behavioral Contract is to increase treatment compliance with the therapeutic regimen, it will be, ideally, tailored to the particular treatment program and designed in collaboration with the clients. This joint effort, established at the outset, provides a sense of teamwork, which, in turn, establishes a cooperative spirit and enhances motivation. Before designing the contract, identify the areas to include and have in mind areas of flexibility (e.g., date at which abstinence must be achieved to continue with treatment) and those areas that are nonnegotiable (e.g., abstinence cannot be downgraded to controlled drinking).

Step 1. Explore the following topics to be included in the Behavioral Contract:

1. The obligations of the counselor, such as preparing homework assignments
2. The obligations of the client, such as completing homework assignments and notifying the therapist when appointments cannot be kept
3. Benefits to be gained if these obligations are fulfilled
4. Methods of evaluating whether or not responsibilities are carried out
5. Consequences for failure to carry out responsibilities
6. Number and frequency of therapy sessions and/or the date on which treatment will be concluded
7. A specific time when progress will be evaluated and the contract renegotiated or treatment terminated (in the case of continued drinking or relapse)

Step 2. Create a clear and detailed contract with clients that includes a description of the out-of-session exercises clients are to be complete. The treatment approach outlined in this book is dependent on clients completing self-monitoring charts between sessions. When a description of required behavior is written specifically, clients are more likely to be clear about what is expected of them and about the program. For example, if requirements regarding the completion of out-of-session exercises are included in the Behavioral Contract at the start of treatment, clients may take the exercises more seriously. Time limits are also important in a contract. People will sometimes be willing to pursue a time-limited goal although they are unwilling to participate in a long-range program.

Step 3. Although therapeutically it is preferable to design the contract with the clients, logistically it is easier to have the contract prepared and ready to sign. If you design the contract with your clients you might type out a general contract, leaving blanks to be filled in during the first session. Another option is to design the contract during the first session, type it up afterwards, and bring it to the following session for everyone to sign. In any event, there need to be three copies, one for each client to take home and one for the therapist. Once the contract is completed, review each item separately so that clients clearly understand each portion of the agreement. Then each member of the treatment signs and dates the contract.

Signing the Behavioral Contract is also a beneficial way to mark the end of the Preparation Phase of treatment and the beginning of the Early Treatment Phase.

For the agreed-upon goals to be achieved, cooperation is required. The signatures below indicate that:

CLIENT AGREES	COUNSELOR AGREES
1. To be abstinent from alcohol and other drugs during the entire treatment program.	1. To attend all 20 sessions. If an emergency arises that necessitates canceling a session, to notify the clients as soon as possible.
2. To attend all 20 sessions. If an emergency arises that necessitates canceling the session, to notify the counselor as soon as possible.	2. To arrive on time and stay the full 90 minutes.
3. To arrive on time and to stay the full 90 minutes.	3. To prepare relevant out-of-session exercises for the clients.
4. To complete out-of-session exercises and bring completed assignments to each session.	

_____   _____
Client   Counselor

_____   _____
Date   Date

COUPLES' ALCOHOLISM TREATMENT
UNIVERSITY OF CALIFORNIA–SANTA BARBARA

FIGURE 3.1. Sample Behavioral Contract.

For the agreed-upon goals to be achieved, cooperation is required. The signatures below indicate that:

CLIENT AGREES	COUNSELOR AGREES
1. To reduce or eliminate _____ during the (target behavior) entire treatment program.	1. To attend all 20 sessions. If an emergency arises that necessitates canceling the session, to notify the clients as soon as possible.
2. To attend all 20 sessions. If an emergency arises that necessitates canceling a session, to notify the counselor as soon as possible.	2. To arrive on time and stay the full 90 minutes.
3. To arrive on time and stay the full 90 minutes.	3. To prepare relevant out-of-session exercises for the clients.
4. To complete out-of-session exercises and bring completed assignments to each session.	

_____   _____
Client   Counselor

_____   _____
Date   Date

COUPLES' ALCOHOLISM TREATMENT
UNIVERSITY OF CALIFORNIA–SANTA BARBARA

FIGURE 3.2. Sample Behavioral Contract.

CHAPTER 4

Phase II:
Early Treatment

Overview

Self-Monitoring: Level I
    ♦ Drinking Chain I and Target Behavior Chart I
Enhancing the Couple's Relationship
    ♦ Pleasant Events

Materials Needed:
    ♦ Drinking Chain I and Target Behavior Chart I (Forms 1 and 2)
    ♦ Two Pleasant Events Schedules (Form 4)
    ♦ Exercise Records (Form 3)
    ♦ Pencils and Clipboards

Recommended number of sessions: 4

Goals: *1. Engage the couple in treatment.*
       2. Teach self-monitoring and begin to understand clients' triggers for drinking and the target behavior.
       3. Introduce the concept of "pleasant events" to enhance the couple's relationship.

The previous chapter included goals in which the primary aim was to introduce the clients to therapy and to begin building a foundation for treatment. The goals in Chapter 4 are aimed at engaging the couple in treatment and beginning therapeutic interventions. The first intervention, self-monitoring, allows the clients and therapist to begin developing a functional analysis of the drinking problem and the problem the partner has chosen to target.

    The second intervention addressed in this chapter is to help the clients enhance their relationship by engaging in pleasant events. Clients are given the opportunity to explore possible pleasant events, to determine which events are enjoyable while sober, and to plan activities with each other that they both find pleasurable. It is also recommended that the communication skills from Chapter 5 be introduced during this phase of treatment.

SELF-MONITORING: LEVEL I

In the beginning of treatment, clients are taught to self-monitor their urges, cravings, and/or thoughts to drink and engage in the target behavior. Introduce the Drinking Chain I and Target Behavior Chart I (Forms 1 and 2) and explain both the purpose and the technique of self-monitoring. It may take a week or two for clients to get the hang of completing the charts and be able to fill them in reliably and in detail.

Rationale

The Drinking Chain I and Target Behavior Chart I are designed to help the clients self-monitor their urges to drink and to engage in the target behavior. Self-monitoring is a well-known cognitive-behavioral strategy and serves to help the clients become aware of their automatic thoughts and behaviors, as well as the consequences of these behaviors. Additionally, these daily records of automatic thoughts help the clients self-monitor affect changes, correctly label emotions, and recognize the relationship between feeling and thinking (Beck et al., 1979).

1. Drinking Chain I and Target Behavior Chart I introduce the concept of "triggers" to the clients and help them begin identifying particular antecedents (i.e., situations, people, thoughts, etc.) to drinking or engaging in the target behavior. Drinking Chain II and Target Behavior Chart II (Forms 6 and 7, introduced later in Chapter 6) help the clients identify their automatic thoughts and feelings that lead to the behavior in focus.

2. These charts are also used for identifying patterns in the clients' drinking and target behaviors. As patterns are recognized, appropriate interventions can be implemented. For example, a pattern may emerge where a client always has an urge to drink right when he or she gets home from work. Thus, an appropriate intervention may involve helping the client deal with the transition from work to home so as to reduce his or her urge to drink.

3. When the clients understand the relationship between thoughts and feelings, they can begin to explore effective coping strategies for dealing with their emotions and disruptive automatic thoughts. Clients will be taught to counter their automatic thoughts with rational thoughts

and try behavioral coping strategies to deal with their emotions, rather than to escape by drinking or engaging in the target behavior.

Procedure

Because the Drinking Chain I and Target Behavior Chart I are central to the therapy program, sufficient time must be allowed to introduce, explain, and practice using them. Proceed slowly, and stop frequently to ask if the material is clear and to ask if the clients have questions. Before moving on, the therapist should be relatively confident that the clients have, at least, a preliminary understanding of how to fill out the charts.

Step 1. Begin by explaining the purpose of the Drinking Chain I and Target Behavior Chart I and how they are to be completed. The charts can be described as graphic aids to gaining control over drinking and target behaviors. All the factors, such as situations, events, people, and times of day that might affect a person's decision to drink or to abstain from alcohol, to engage in a target behavior or not, are identified and recorded. By examining the information on the charts it will be possible to identify events that trigger unwanted behavior and to discover patterns to those events. Then more adaptive ways of coping can be determined.

It is not too soon to begin suggesting that the clients' drinking and engagement in the target behavior are voluntary; thus, drinking or engaging in the target behavior are termed "choices" or "decisions" that the clients make. It is also important to begin early in the program to train clients not to view situations as the "cause" of their thoughts, behavior, urges, or feelings; begin by being careful to speak of situations as "triggers" rather than "reasons" or "causes."

Step 2. Column by column, review both charts by using the examples provided on the Drinking Chain I and the Target Behavior Chart I (Forms 1 and 2). Explain that the first column is used to record the day and time of two possible occurrences: when the client experienced an urge to drink or engage in the target behavior, but resisted that urge; or when the client actually did drink or engage in the target behavior. Not uncommon is the client who does not understand what an "urge" is. The therapist might define the word as "a feeling or thought that a person would like to drink," explaining that it could be a physical feeling, an image, or simply a thought. Sometimes clients will deny a desire to drink or engage in the target behavior, but acknowledge thoughts about the behavior. If this occurs, it is *not* important that the client be pinned down until he or she admits to a desire to drink or perform the target behavior; simply use the term "thought" and continue with the exercise.

The second column, "situation," includes *where* the client was, *what* he or she was doing, and *who* was present. The third column is for recording the "trigger," that is, the crucial event that was the stimulus for the client to change a decision to stay sober into a choice to drink, or a decision to abstain from the target behavior into a choice to engage in the behavior. For now it might be easiest to look at what happened immediately before the client began to drink or noticed that he or she felt like drinking. Give a number of examples of triggers, in addition to those included on the charts, explaining that sometimes all that is necessary to trigger an urge to drink is seeing alcohol, passing by a favorite bar, or smelling the scent of beer. In the same way, watching someone light a cigarette can trigger smoking and smelling coffee brewing can trigger an urge for caffeine. Sometimes the trigger is not obviously related to alcohol or to the target behavior. Any stimulus that the client regards as a stressor can trigger the unwanted coping device, such as an argument, changed duties at work, an acquaintance making an insulting remark, or a small inconvenience that feels like a last straw. (Refer to Appendix 2, Exploring Triggers, for additional strategies to help clients who are having difficulty understanding this concept.)

The fourth column is used to record the decision to drink or not, to abstain from the target behavior or not. There are only two possible entries, "Yes" or "No." Because the goal of the treatment for the alcoholic is abstinence, any alcohol, even a sip, should be recorded as a "Yes." In the fifth column, "results," the client describes what happened after he or she made the choice to drink or to abstain, to engage in the target behavior or not. If the client decided to drink, then he or she would record what happened after the decision was made, as well as how much alcohol (in ounces) was consumed. The same would apply to the partner regarding the engagement in the target behavior. If the client decided not to drink, or not to engage in the targeted behavior then what the client did instead should be recorded.

Step 3. When all five columns on the chart have been examined, ask the alcoholic for a recent occurrence when he or she had no intention of drinking yet ended up doing so. Ask the partner for a recent example of a situation in which he or she engaged in the target behavior. Then have both clients fill in their charts with these recent examples and go over their entries; answer questions and help clients with columns that prove to be more difficult for them.

In order to be useful, the information clients present on the charts must be both complete and specific. Many clients have great difficulty being precise. Sometimes clients leave blank the day and time or indicate the day but omit the time, so that we know the incident occurred on

Wednesday, but have no idea at what time of day or night. Often clients do not make the situation column sufficiently clear to get a picture of what happened; for example, the reader does not know exactly where they were or what they were doing. Sometimes important information is omitted; for example, one client failed to note that he had been accompanied by two friends the previous Friday night when he consumed 72 ounces of beer. If the therapist had not questioned the client directly, the missing information would have been misleading in the search for trigger patterns. In this particular case, the presence of friends was important because the friends were old "drinking buddies" the client had managed to avoid until this Friday evening. What clients report on their charts needs to be comprehensive and clear enough for the therapist to visualize the scene.

Also difficult for many clients is the trigger column; most often it is not only specificity that is the problem but also an inability to determine what the trigger might have been. The client should be taught that if identifying what happened immediately before an urge to drink does not elicit the trigger, it is often possible to work back in time through a chain of events until a circumstance earlier in the day, or even earlier in the week, is found that might have led to the trigger.

Step 4. Specify that there is no correct number of entries; some days they might have many entries and some days they might have very few. What is important is that the client record any and all urges (or thoughts) to drink or engage in the target behavior and any and all drinking or target behavior episodes. Request that if there comes a day when the clients had no relevant urges or behavior that they record on the chart a general evaluation of the day, significant events that occurred, and emotional reactions to those events. If clients must write something on the chart, they are less likely to overlook pertinent urges than if they had license to leave days blank. Additionally, important information is often acquired on days when the clients have no urges or thoughts to drink or engage in the target behavior.

Step 5. Alternative Intervention. With clients that appear to have particular difficulty recording their drinking cravings or thoughts to drink and/or engage in the target behavior, it may be helpful to focus on one particular column each session, for the next few sessions. For example, after explaining the charts thoroughly and having the clients practice with examples from their recent past, go back over the examples, paying particular attention to the situation column. You may need to prompt the clients with questions regarding where they were; who they were with; what was happening before, during, and after the urge or thought to drink or engage in the target behavior. Ask the clients to include all of this information in their charts when they complete them each day. Also explain the purpose of this detail; that is, you are looking for patterns that may emerge over time from which you may choose to make specific interventions. For example, if a common situation arises where the client considers drinking after work with two of his work buddies, then this will be an important situation to consider when introducing cognitive and behavioral strategies to deal with the urges.

Reviewing Charts

It is recommended that clients complete the charts daily. Thus, if the therapist and clients are meeting twice weekly, the clients should have at least a couple days' entries between sessions. The following describes how to review the Drinking Chain I and Target Behavior Chart I with clients, which can be done at the beginning of each session throughout the early and middle phases of treatment.

Step 1. Start with one client and first look over the chart for completeness (i.e., was the chart filled in every day and were details in each column provided?). Address any missing days, blank columns, or vague entries.

Step 2. Go over each entry and help the client add whatever detail is necessary in order to give a complete picture of the situation recorded. If the therapist is utilizing the Alternative Intervention suggested above (Step 5), the first session following the introduction of the Drinking Chain I and Target Behavior Chart I may focus on the detail recorded in the situation column. Then, in the following sessions, focus on the trigger column and the results column, respectively.

Step 3. Discuss any entries where the client had an urge and chose to drink or engage in the target behavior. Use the chart to help identify triggers for the drinking episode or engagement in the target behavior. Help the clients determine which areas they may have had control over in changing the stimulus that led them to engage in the drinking and/or target behavior. For example, for clients who routinely drink after work, they could not change the time of day (Column 1); however, they could have possibly changed the situation (Column 2) by going to a sober friend's house directly after work, or going to the gym before going home. Another example, considering the partner this time, could be that the trigger (Column 3) for engaging in the target behavior (eating sweets) was opening the freezer and seeing a pint of ice cream. At this point in the session, the therapist should have the partner explore alternative ways he or she could have handled the urge, without eating the ice cream. Also, the therapist should encourage the alcoholic client and the partner to help brainstorm alternative coping behaviors for each other.

Step 4. Acknowledge any entries where the client had an urge and chose *not* to drink or engage in the target behavior. Explore at some length how he or she dealt with the urge and felt about the successful intervention. As the clients' responses are discussed in the case where they chose to abstain, ask if there is anything they feel they "miss out on" as a result of choosing not to drink or to engage in the target behavior. For example, one woman whose target behavior was abstaining from sweets expressed a concern about missing out on rewards for work accomplished; it was important to explore ways, other than eating sweets, that she could reward herself. Another example is that of a male alcoholic who was troubled about missing out on socializing with his work buddies; it was important to explore ways to socialize with friends from work and still remain abstinent. For most clients there is a feeling of missing out on something or a feeling of loss that goes along with cessation of drinking or engaging in a target behavior. It is important to explore this reaction, normalize the feelings, and discuss coping strategies to deal with the loss.

Step 5. Explore the types of behaviors the clients perform after they decide to drink or not, to engage in the target behavior or not. Discuss which of these behaviors are effective coping strategies, reinforcing of abstinence; if necessary, explore alternative coping strategies. Time permitting, begin to consider the cognitive strategies that clients use when coping with urges to drink and engage in the target behavior. Ask if clients notice any patterns, not only within the results column, but also between each situation and the respective result, between each trigger and the respective result. Make note of these emerging patterns. For example, a pattern might emerge in the results column indicating that a client's only coping strategy to deal with urges to drink is to become angry and start an argument; and, by looking at the situation column, it becomes clear that these arguments occur every Wednesday after the client has worked a 12-hour day. Thus, the therapist is gathering information that will be helpful in deciding what interventions will be most useful for each individual client. This client, for example, will need help discovering and implementing coping strategies for (1) recognizing the trigger, (2) dealing with stress, and perhaps, (3) reducing his or her workload.

Step 6. If there is time, go over every entry on each client's chart; if not, go over as many as possible and look for any emerging patterns. Bring these patterns to the client's attention and/or ask the clients if they notice any patterns and make note of them on the charts.

Step 7. When reviewing the partner's Target Behavior Chart, there is an ideal opportunity to elicit feedback regarding how similar and/or different abstaining from the target behavior is to abstaining from alcohol, and vice versa. This is also an ideal time to begin eliciting empathy and understanding from the partner regarding the recovery process, as well as to begin reinforcing the alcoholic's support of the partner.

Exercises

1. Have both clients complete the charts each day.

2. Discuss when the clients plan on completing their charts each day and explore ways to make the task more convenient for each of them. If it is helpful, use an Exercise Record (see Form 3) to help clients remember their assignments. Remind them to bring the charts in each time you meet. We suggest having clients complete charts throughout the early and middle phases of treatment. It is in these stages of treatment that self-monitoring is most helpful. When clients begin to move into the later phases of treatment, it is important to focus on out-of-session exercises that will be helpful in preventing relapse, and have a greater likelihood of being continued after treatment ends. Although clients often report that the self-monitoring is very helpful, they are quite happy either to quit monitoring altogether or to reduce their monitoring to once a week, primarily because it is a labor intensive, time-consuming exercise.

3. When assigning exercises to complete the charts this first time, stress the importance of thorough information, advise clients to include on their charts every urge to drink or engage in the target behavior, and provide them with extra charts in case they run out of space. Next, explain the importance of recording an urge as soon as it occurs and suggest that they carry their charts with them during the day so that they will not forget. Most clients, however, object to doing this because it is inconvenient and because others might observe them. A second choice would be to put the charts in one place where they will always be sure to find them and to fill out the chart daily, building it into the day's routine. Work with the clients until each has identified the best time and place to complete their charting.

4. Refer to the Compliance Enhancers (Appendix 3) for clients who are having difficulty completing out-of-session assignments.

Case Illustration: Charting

Beth completes her Target Behavior Chart I daily and includes detailed accounts of her thoughts about using caffeine. She has one incident where she had a cola drink (target behavior: abstain from caffeine) and her entry regarding this incident is less detailed than her other accounts. Mike's charting is not as consistent. He has one detailed entry the first time he drank, followed by a vague entry for the second drinking day, and somewhat vague entries for other, nondrinking days. Because Mike had two drinking episodes, the therapist decides to review Mike's Drinking Chain I before Beth's Target Behavior Chart I. Mike is able to identify the time, date, situation, and trigger for his drinking. He was coming home from work on a Friday evening when he remembered that he had left his paycheck on his desk. He returned to work and, paycheck in hand, ran into a friend who invited him to "Happy Hour." Mike has entered "stress," "frustration at not being able to ever drink again" and "paycheck in hand" in the trigger column. He reports that he didn't think a lot about whether he should or should not drink, and just went with his friend to a local bar. He has entered in the results and alternatives column that he drank five beers, drove home, and avoided Beth until she finally discovered that he had been drinking. Mike has not entered any "alternatives" on his chart. His second drinking entry occurred the next day when he was feeling so guilty about drinking that he "went ahead and drank some more." This second entry is less detailed than the first.

The therapist first explores with Mike what happened on the second drinking day, having him fill in his chart in more detail. The trigger on the second day was an argument he had with Beth about the previous night of drinking. After reviewing both incidents, the therapist asks both Mike and Beth if they notice any similarities in the drinking episodes. Beth points out that Mike drank around 6:00 P.M. on both nights and that he drank with his friend Paul on both occasions. Mike realizes that he felt "bad" on both occasions–stressed on the first night, mad and guilty on the second night. The therapist then has the couple brainstorm alternatives together for Mike in both cases; that is, how he could have dealt with the stress on the Friday, and how could he have dealt with his guilt and anger on next night. The therapist also explores why the "paycheck in hand" is a trigger and how Mike could have dealt with this differently.

Lastly, the therapist helps Mike explore the nondrinking days in more detail to determine what was happening such that he was able to remain abstinent. For the most part, Mike realizes that when he is busy, feels good about himself, and is not arguing with Beth, he has few thoughts about drinking. The therapist emphasizes the behaviors in which Mike engaged when he thought about drinking, but refrained from doing so (e.g., took the dog for a walk, watched TV, and went for a run).

The therapist then discusses Beth's chart with the couple, reviewing all entries in order. Beth justifies drinking cola, rather than coffee, because it has "less caffeine." Mike promptly confronts her on her rationalization and her agreement of quitting *all* caffeine. At first Beth is defensive and the therapist points out that this would be like Mike drinking beer instead of a mixed drink and asks her how she would feel about this switch of beverages. Beth is able to see the parallel and laughs at her initial justification. Both partners begin to see the benefit of participating together in this manner. The therapist also notes that Mike readily challenged Beth, but did not offer any supportive feedback. The therapist is able to pull Mike into the discussion by asking him to help Beth think of alternative ways she could have dealt with her desire to drink caffeine when she was tired and had to work 5 more hours.

The couple agree to continue charting. Beth is to focus on coming up with alternative behaviors in which to engage when she is tired and to include detail in her charting regardless of whether she drinks caffeine or not. Mike is also to focus on finding alternative behaviors when he is not feeling good and to be more detailed in his nondrinking entries. Both partners are encouraged to ask each other for support in coming up with alternative coping strategies.

Note. At this phase of treatment, it is not unusual to have clients drink or engage in the target behavior. However, continued drinking or engagement in the target behavior needs to be addressed and goals of treatment reviewed.

ENHANCING THE COUPLE'S RELATIONSHIP

The Pleasant Events Schedule (PES; Form 4) is introduced as a tool to help couples find enjoyable activities to do together while remaining abstinent and unengaged in the target behavior. Having enjoyable activities to do by oneself, as well as with one's partner, is an important foundation for an alcoholic to build in early recovery.

Rationale

For most couples, when alcohol has become a problem for one or both of the partners, the relationship suffers significantly. They no longer participate in the activities they once enjoyed, often for fear that the alcoholic will become intoxicated, embarrass the family, or become withdrawn or abusive. Hobbies, sports, and other interests often take a back seat to trying to keep the family together, the bills paid, and the alcoholic out of trouble. Consequently, when a couple comes into treatment, it is not surprising when they report that they have not done anything "fun" together for a long time—perhaps years. If they are having fun with each other, or more likely, with their drinking buddies, the activities usually involve alcohol or the target behavior. Therefore, the idea of "pleasant events" may initially be met with resistance; however, our experience indicates that for most clients it eventually becomes a highlight of the program.

1. Having couples go on "dates," begin a new hobby, or simply spend time *together,* is a common practice in couple therapy. In behavioral couple therapy with alcoholic clients, Barbara McCrady (1989) introduced the idea of "Love Days" for the purpose of providing couples with an opportunity to experience more pleasurable time together and to interact more positively at home.

2. The original PES, a 320-item list of potentially enjoyable activities, was developed by MacPhillamy and Lewinsohn (1982) to assist in the treatment of depression. It is based on the theory that depressed people do not receive adequate reinforcement in their lives and that by increasing their level of pleasant activities, they can control their depression. The PES is used to identify events the client enjoys, to assess the client's rate of pleasant activities, and to evaluate how much pleasure the client is deriving from those activities.

3. The PES was adapted for use with alcoholics by eliminating seven items dealing with alcohol, drugs, and tobacco; eliminating items that did not appear to be pleasant activities; adding three blank lines for clients to fill in their own pleasant activities; eliminating the frequency count; and instructing clients first to rate items they find pleasurable, then go back over the list to check items they find pleasurable when sober.

4. In addition to being of benefit to the couple, the PES can be used by the clients individually. For many alcoholics, activities have become so narrow that when asked why they drink, they respond, "because I'm bored," or, "because there is nothing else to do." And, in fact, what they say is true, because alcoholic clients have become so used to drinking during most, if not all, activities, that when alcohol is unavailable, they are at a loss to find something else to do. Often, when clients come back after completing the PES, they will comment on the number of activities they remembered having enjoyed in the past, or how many activities they had never thought of doing but might like to do.

5. The PES is also appropriate for the partner in abstaining from the target behavior. As with alcohol, a target behavior can be a substitute for an emotionally unavailable partner and become a part of most of the person's activities. For example, one partner whose target behavior was snacking between meals, found that a great many of her activities—reading, watching television, being with friends–involved eating. The PES was used to help her find enjoyable activities that did not involve eating.

Procedure

Before introducing the PES, take some time to explore with the clients what they currently do "for fun" and what is pleasurable to each individually, as well as together. Also inquire about what they have done together in the past that they both found enjoyable. Then introduce the PES and the rationale behind incorporating it in the treatment. The instructions are self-explanatory, but take some time to go over the PES and make sure both clients are clear about how to complete the form, including going back over the form and marking items that would be pleasurable while abstaining from alcohol. If the partner's target behavior is appropriate for this exercise, he or she can mark which items would be pleasurable while abstaining from the targeted behavior as well.

Exercise

We suggest that the clients complete the PES individually and refrain from sharing their responses with each other until the next session. Explain to the clients that during the next session, they will be asked to review the forms together and will choose one event to do together during the following week. Let the clients know that the PES takes about 1 hour to complete and encourage them to set aside time where they will not be disrupted in order to give their full attention to the task.

Review of Exercise

Step 1. When reviewing the PES with clients, find out what is pleasurable to each client, independent of the partner, and then explore what commonalities exist between them. Focus on the items rated "1" and "2," that is, items rated somewhat or very pleasant. In addition, concentrate on items in Column S, that is, those items that are enjoyable when the client is abstinent from alcohol or the target behavior.

Step 2. It may also be helpful to explore those items that the clients find enjoyable only while under the influence or while engaged in the target behavior and briefly discuss the possible loss associated with cessation of these activities.

Step 3. When working with the couple to determine what commonalities exist on their forms, focus only on the "2's" that are enjoyable during abstinence for both of them. Have each client discuss what is pleasurable in that particular activity. If no commonalities exist with the "2" responses, move to the "1's" and look for commonalities; if none are present, take time to find an activity the couple enjoys doing together, even though it is not on the PES, and add that activity to the end of the PES.

Step 4. When the commonalities have been highlighted, ask the clients to choose *one* that they are willing to do together during the next week. Have them start out with an activity that is the least threatening to abstinence and has the greatest likelihood of success. Inquire how the clients feel about doing this activity together, and explore positive or negative feelings associated with the activity. It is not uncommon for clients to feel excitement, discomfort, or fear, or to be hesitant to commit to an activity lest their partner back out of the agreement. Discuss any time constraints or other obstacles. Finally, explain that they will be given the opportunity to continue to choose different pleasant events each week throughout the remainder of the program.

Step 5. Help clients problem solve any difficulties they may have with completing this task (e.g., difficulties agreeing on an event, one partner forgetting or being late to the event, or child care). After the couple completes a pleasant event, review how the exercise went for them. Do not assume the couple was abstinent or that alcohol and/or other drugs were absent from the event. Spending "fun" time together while abstinent may be a big step for some couples and they may have difficulty with this exercise in the beginning of treatment. Inquire whether alcohol or other drugs were present and, if so, why? If not, ask how the event was and how the couple felt being abstinent. Inquire whether this activity enhanced their relationship and whether it was reinforcing of sobriety.

Note. Some couples are still very angry and resentful of one another in early treatment and spending time together can be difficult. If this is the case, encourage clients to use their communication skills (discussed in Chapter 5) to begin to work through anger and resentment. Referring clients to individual therapy and/or support groups, in addition to the couple therapy, is another alternative to dealing with a couple who is having a difficult time letting go of the anger, hurt, and so forth in this focused treatment approach.

Step 6. Have the couple complete a new pleasant event weekly or at least once a month and review each time.

Case Illustration: Pleasant Events

As with many couples who are presenting for couple therapy and/or alcoholism treatment, Mike and Beth report that it has been a long time since they spent any time together doing an enjoyable activity. Beth readily asserts that this is the case because of Mike's drinking. Mike, however, claims that this had been a problem even a few years back when he was drinking very little. Again, the split between the couple with respect to their views on the source of problems surfaces. That is, Beth sees most of the problems as related to Mike's drinking, while Mike sees most of the problems as related to other circumstances. The therapist points this issue out to the couple and gives both partners feedback. On the one hand, Beth's continual pointing of the finger appears to be reinforcing Mike's defensiveness and denial about his drinking problem. On the other hand, Mike's continual minimization of his drinking problem, and in particular the consequences on his family, reinforces Beth's need to convince him of his problem. (Note: Part of the therapist's responsibility is to help the couple identify those behaviors that are reinforcing of abstinence and those that are reinforcing of the drinking or drinking lifestyle.)

When the couple is able to recognize that they both contribute to the problems they are experiencing, the therapist moves on. The couple has completed their individual PES and, in session, explores the "2's" that they both have (i.e., the events they find the most enjoyable). It turns out that the couple have quite a few "2's" in common that they enjoyed doing together sober, including such activities as, "camping," "cooking," "kissing," "bicycling," and "talking about their jobs." The couple discusses that these were activities they used to do together when they were first dating and early in their marriage. They choose two activities to complete over the next 2 weeks, including "camping" and "bicycling." In addition, the couple has previously discussed having a dissatisfying sex life and agree that they would like to start improving this area of their relationship slowly by just being more affectionate with each other. Beth notes during this discussion that a "benefit" for her from Mike's drinking is that she does not have to deal with her fears of intimacy that have surfaced as a result of her abusive first marriage. This realization leads into the second part of the discussion regarding fears and fantasies that the couple have about spending time together.

Note. If the couple does not complete the pleasant event, it may be necessary to explore the fears they may be experiencing in greater detail. For example, a spouse might fear that her husband will drink or that she might disappoint him. If this is the case, it is important to have the couple choose nonthreatening events with which to start.

CHAPTER 5

Communication Skills Training

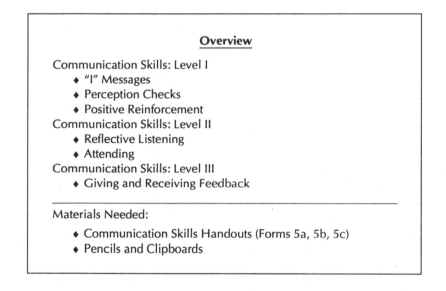

Overview

Communication Skills: Level I
- ♦ "I" Messages
- ♦ Perception Checks
- ♦ Positive Reinforcement

Communication Skills: Level II
- ♦ Reflective Listening
- ♦ Attending

Communication Skills: Level III
- ♦ Giving and Receiving Feedback

Materials Needed:

- ♦ Communication Skills Handouts (Forms 5a, 5b, 5c)
- ♦ Pencils and Clipboards

Recommended number of sessions: to be incorporated throughout treatment

Goals: 1. Teach clients effective communication skills.
2. Give clients tools for enhancing their relationship.

Helping clients build a foundation together from which they can support their abstinence is a critical step in the early phases of couple therapy. By learning basic communication skills, the clients' relationship can be enhanced, their ability to develop support systems can be strengthened, and their ability to deal with high-risk situations can be improved.

COMMUNICATION SKILLS: LEVEL I
Rationale

Research has shown that many alcoholics have inadequate communication skills (Marlatt & Gordon, 1985). This is often the case with a client who grew up in an alcoholic family where he or she was never taught how to express feelings, problem solve, deal with criticism, or work through arguments. Moreover, a client who was taught these skills growing up may have forgotten how to implement them as a result of long-term drinking. The consequence in either case is unsatisfactory relationships and poor coping strategies to deal with feelings such as frustration and anger that naturally arise in interpersonal relationships.

1. In this initial level of skills training, we emphasize three communication skills: (1) clear expression of feelings through "I" messages, (2) perception checks, and (3) positive reinforcement. If the clients can grasp these communication skills, they often see improvements in their relationship and are able to support each other much more effectively. We recognize that many clients need additional communication skills to help strengthen their sobriety and prevent relapse.

2. Although couples often realize that they do not communicate well, they frequently do not fully appreciate the extent of the damage done to their relationship by maladaptive styles of interaction and may need to be sold on the importance of making considerable effort to change the way they speak to each other. To help clients learn the value of changing their communication patterns, it is helpful to initiate a brief discussion about how they typically express or fail to express various feelings (both positive and negative) and what the results of such expression tend to be. One might, for example, ask how they communicate anger, and elicit the troublesome aspects of this communication, such as blaming, name calling, generalizing, arguing about who is right, storing up resentment and then exploding, threatening, and so on. Labeling such a style as a habit or pattern that has been learned and can, with effort, be unlearned tends to defuse some of the feelings clients may have of failure, inadequacy or blame. The sequence of responses and the inevitable outcome of these destructive types of communication can be elicited, until both clients understand clearly that the major effect of their current communication style is that each partner ends up feeling not understood and not accepted by the other and that intimacy is thus reduced. This introduction sets the stage for clients to appreciate the need for improved communication in the interest of a more satisfactory and harmonious relationship.

Procedure

If substantive change is to occur in clients' communication styles, skills must initially be treated as separate entities, to be modeled, taught, and practiced under supervision as individual units. The process of skill acquisition often begins with the use of a simple formula that clients may find unnatural, even aversive. They need to be reassured that breaking old habits often feels uncomfortable at first but that after a little practice of the basic skill, they will develop a more personal and individual style and will quickly learn how to integrate the various skills. The skills to be taught are expressing one's own feelings clearly, expressing the impact of the other's behavior on oneself, checking out one's perception of the other's state of mind, reflecting back both the content and feelings in the other person's statement, and responding to perceived criticism by the other person. All these are to be accomplished without the addition of destructive or manipulative material. With some clients, especially those unaccustomed to clarity of expression or unused to identifying emotions, the therapist may need to break each skill into smaller components, model each step, and provide considerable feedback on the clients' practice. More verbal or more introspective clients may require less directiveness initially, but must still be persuaded of the necessity for practice. In order to practice these skills in vivo, help the clients to establish times and safe topics. Some clients find it helpful, for example, to set aside 15 minutes when they first meet at the end of the day. Others may find another time easier.

Skill 1: "I" Messages—Expressing One's Own Feelings Clearly

Clients need to understand that most communications (and particularly the ones that tend to lead to fights, misunderstandings, or hurt feelings) contain both factual information and feelings. Sometimes, this two-part message is not very clear, which makes it difficult for the listener to understand exactly what is being communicated. A first step, then, is to state the message clearly. Like all skills, this will need to be practiced until it replaces the old habit, so clients can be encouraged to begin their practice with the simple I-message formula:

"I feel Y when X," or, "When X happens, I feel Y."

Step 1. Begin by asking each client in turn to complete a number of feeling stems (e.g., "I feel angry when . . ."; "I feel excited when . . ."), making sure to include both *positive and negative* emotions. At this point, neither person should respond to what the other says.

If the couple engages in frequent conflict or each tends to see criticism or blame in almost anything the other says, then the therapist should instruct the couple to use examples that are *not* related to their life together; for example, "I feel angry when the traffic backs up and I am late for work." This kind of simple direct statement is quite foreign to many people, so the therapist might want to ask clients for feedback on any difficulty they are experiencing. One quite common reaction, especially for clients from families where emotion was not expressed or where the expression of emotion was punished, is to feel exposed and vulnerable to attack by the partner even when disclosing apparently innocuous feelings. For such clients, one effect of this exercise is to begin the process of desensitization to the expression of feelings.

Step 2. When clients are reasonably adept at producing simple "I" statements, practice can be extended to messages that refer to the partner's behavior, using the following formula:

"When you _____ [behavior], I feel _____ [emotion] because _____ [specific reason]."

Or start with the emotion, as in:

"I feel _____ [emotion] when you _____ [behavior] because _____ [specific reason]."

An example of the above message would be, "When you promise to be home at six and then arrive two hours late, I feel angry because the dinner I worked so hard to prepare is invariably ruined."

It is important that both partners select relatively nonthreatening topics for this practice, and that positive as well as negative feelings be included. Clients should again take turns in this exercise, simply listening to each other without responding. During this exercise, partners often become upset because they perceive themselves to be attacked, criticized, or manipulated by what they are hearing. Encourage them to regard the partner's statement as simple information about the partner's state of mind, and reassure them both that they will eventually learn how to respond to perceived criticism or attack. Remind them that for now the task is for both of them to learn how to communicate their experiences and to listen without judgment, not to decide the justice or truth of that experience. As in Step 1, the exercise should be thoroughly debriefed for feelings of discomfort and anxiety.

Skill 2: Perception Checks

Explain the concept of "perception checks" and give examples. One of the ways in which a couple's communication wreaks havoc with their relationship is when one partner interprets the motivation or intentions of the other. An example of this ineffective communication is when one partner says to the other, "The reason you bought that bottle of bourbon was to get even with me for yelling at your mother." It is often the case that we have mistaken views of what another person is feeling or thinking. A perception check is a simple yet highly effective communication technique that involves (1) identifying what you noticed, (2) stating your guess as to what that behavior means, and then (3) asking if your interpretation is accurate.

Step 1. After reviewing the concept of perception checks, have clients consider the following examples:

"Your voice got very loud when you talked about Bill, and I wonder if you're going to lose your temper and start hitting someone."

"You seem to be unusually quiet. Are you not feeling well?" "I noticed that you frowned when I was talking with Ralph and I thought you were judging me. Was I wrong?"

The key to a good perception check is simply to *ask* if one's perception of the other's behavior is correct, not to *assume* that it is.

Step 2. Prepare several practice situations, each on a separate 3 × 5 card. Here are some possible situations:

1. For the past 30 minutes your partner has been preparing dinner and in the process making a good deal of noise, banging cupboards and pots.
2. Last night your partner went to bed at 8 P.M. and slept this morning until 9 A.M.
3. You have a new friend, Leslie. The past several times you mentioned Leslie, your partner has become very quiet.

Step 3. Have clients take turns responding with perception checks to two or three of these practice situations.

Step 4. Next, ask clients to identify and write situations of their own; again, have clients take turns responding with perception checks to these new situations.

Exercises

Give clients Communication Skills: Level I Handouts (Forms 5a, 5b) and
have them practice the exercises at home.

Skill 3: Positive Reinforcement

Most people begin relationships because doing so is rewarding and
because the partner is a source of reinforcement for them. Often, for a
variety of reasons, and especially when alcohol is involved, the rewarding
aspects of the relationship are forgotten and only the unpleasant facets of
the partnership seem to be present. It is not uncommon for couples to
come into treatment thinking nothing positive at all about one another.
To make matters worse, even when people do have positive thoughts about
one another, they often do not express those thoughts aloud.

Step 1. The first step in teaching the clients to reinforce one another
is to explain the value of reinforcement; that is, positive reinforcement
feels good, makes for a pleasant atmosphere in the relationship, increases
the probability that people will continue doing what is being reinforced,
and strengthens the partnership.

Step 2. Sometimes simply reminding clients to reward one another
is sufficient. However, sometimes it is necessary to help clients view their
partners in positive terms so that they will be able to think of something
positive to say. To do this, it is useful to ask each partner, in turn, what it
was about the other that was originally attractive to them. Another
method is to acknowledge that there was some connection between the
partners that brought them into treatment together and to explore what
this connection might be.

Step 3. Encourage clients to give each other positive reinforcement for
the behavior changes they are making in and out of therapy. These rewards
can be in the form of either verbal or nonverbal messages; smiles, compliments, hugs, or doing something nice for the other person are all positive
rewards. Teach the clients to be *specific* about why they are offering the
rewards. For example, when giving a compliment, clients should be specific
about what behavior they are pleased with. A person might say, "You look
nice today with your new hairstyle," or, "I have noticed that since you
stopped drinking, you have been dressing up more often and look very
attractive." An example of a nonverbal reward would be for the alcoholic
to make a nice meal for the partner. It would also be beneficial for the
alcoholic to offer a verbal statement letting his partner know why he made

the nice meal. He could say, for example, "I made dinner this evening because I appreciate your participation in therapy with me." When hugging, or showing affection, a person might add, "That particular hug is because I feel very proud of you for having 12 days of sobriety."

Step 4. After explaining positive reinforcement to clients, ask them how often they currently offer this kind of reward to each other. Explore what the possible benefits are if they begin to communicate appreciation for one another more directly and more frequently. Also, explore any fears or concerns the clients have in initiating this type of communication. A common concern was voiced by a partner in treatment with his alcoholic wife: "Last time I commented on my wife's sobriety, she went out and drank and I felt disappointed and foolish." If such concerns arise, this is a good opportunity to explore how the partner has given feedback in the past and if there are more effective ways to express appreciation. Additionally, the couple's fears of the alcoholic returning to drinking and their questions regarding how they should respond, is an important topic that needs to be addressed.

Step 5. Two strategies for helping clients get started giving each other positive reinforcement are (1) to have them ask each other what types of things they appreciate being noticed and (2) to give each other feedback regarding the most effective way to state the positive reinforcement. For example, one partner might say, "I appreciate it when you notice that I have cleaned the house," and, "I think it is helpful when you give me compliments directly, rather than just praising me to others."

Step 6. Another strategy that may be helpful for clients who are having a difficult time letting go of resentments, is to have them utilize the following formula, giving one "resentment" and two "appreciations" to one another:

"I resent you for _____ ."
"I appreciate you for _____ ."
"I appreciate you for _____ ."

Step 7. Have couples practice this exercise in the present session and in subsequent sessions, as well as at home. *Make sure to notice when clients give each other spontaneous positive reinforcement and acknowledge this behavior.* If, in future sessions, clients do not appear to be offering each other positive reinforcement, discuss what might be getting in the way of implementing this skill and help clients work through these obstacles.

COMMUNICATION SKILLS: LEVEL II

A second type of skill that is critical for effective communication between a couple is "active listening." The skills involved in actively listening may be particularly difficult for the couple who have "tuned each other out" for a long time and selectively listen to what one another is saying. Active listening, which involves the two skills introduced below, reflective listening and attending, can be very beneficial for clients to master.

Skill 1: Reflective Listening

Reflective listening is perhaps the most difficult communication skill, requiring the most self-control, objectivity, and empathy.

Step 1. Explain the purpose of reflective listening and give examples. Explain to clients that, in order to feel accepted and understood, the speaker must know that the listener has heard both the thoughts and the feelings being expressed. Even if a person does not agree with a statement, it is important to convey that he or she has at least understood it. Again, this style of communication feels quite foreign at first and it is easy to slip back into old habits; thus, clients can be encouraged to use formulas in the early stages of practicing this skill.

The formula that follows may be helpful:

"What I hear you saying is _____ [paraphrase content and reflect emotion]."

For example:

SPEAKER: "I can't stand the way you leave your books all over the living room."

LISTENER: "What I hear you saying is that you feel annoyed with the way I mess up the living room," or, "You are saying that when I leave my stuff all over, you get mad at me," or, "What I hear you saying is that you are angry with my messiness."

It may be necessary to spend some time with clients helping them grasp the concepts of "paraphrasing content" and "reflecting feelings." Many clients have a difficult time concisely reflecting back to their partners the thoughts and feelings expressed without adding their own edits and interpretations.

Step 2. Point out to clients that simply acknowledging the other person's state of mind does not necessarily mean that one is agreeing with that point of view, or giving in, or allowing oneself to be manipulated, or any other fears that the listener may have.

Step 3. One effective way to demonstrate both the skill itself and the powerful effect of reflective listening is for the therapist to practice active listening with each client for a few minutes as the client tells a story with some emotional impact. Clients can then take turns listening to each other, with corrective feedback from the therapist. To enhance the focus on skill acquisition, help clients to choose topics that will not lead to overwhelming emotional arousal.

Step 4. After each episode of listening, elicit feedback from the speaker about the experience of being truly listened to. This generally provides considerable reinforcement for the listener who has been struggling to practice the skill.

Exercise

Discuss with the clients which communication skill would be most beneficial for them to practice first. Help them come up with an assignment that will allow them to practice this skill at home. As treatment progresses, have clients continue to practice and master all of these communication skills. Give clients Communication Skills: Level II Handout (Form 5c) to take home. If using the Exercise Records, remind the clients to write this assignment down on their records.

Review of Exercise

Along with the clients, decide how much time will be devoted to reviewing these skills during therapy sessions. As skills are reviewed, help clients with difficulties and continually encourage them to utilize these skills in session. Reinforce the use of communication skills by acknowledging clients when they have used skills appropriately in session. Give homework exercises as necessary.

Skill 2: Attending

The final communication skill to be taught at this level of the treatment program is "attending." Employing appropriate attending skills is an important responsibility of any listener. These skills, including attentive body posture, minimal body movement, eye contact, and arrangement of a nondistracting environment, indicate that the listener is paying careful attention (Bolton, 1979).

Step 1. Merely reviewing with clients how attending skills can help facilitate communication and how nonattending habits can thwart communication may be beneficial. Once clients are reminded of these skills, they will often begin to attend to each other more fully and request that their partner do the same. Many couples have the habit of talking about important matters while simultaneously watching television, reading the newspaper, or engaging in some other activity. Ask about the frequency of misunderstandings and/or feelings of being ignored as a result of nonattending habits. This inquiry may help to reinforce the benefits of practicing these skills. Additionally, the therapist can explore with the couple other areas of their lives where they may find these skills particularly helpful (e.g., at work or with their children).

Step 2. As with all communication skills, be sensitive to the clients' cultural background when introducing these attending behaviors. Specific "habits" that appear ineffectual (e.g., avoiding eye contact) may be appropriate and consistent with a client's cultural upbringing. It is critical to explore, and to be sensitive to, these factors in order to build rapport with clients and maximize treatment outcome.

Step 3. The following exercises may be helpful for clients who are unfamiliar with attending skills and/or need practice. The exercises also include practice of reflective listening skills.

Round 1

1. Have clients sit across from each other and choose a *nonthreatening* topic to discuss (e.g., their ideal vacation).
2. Explain that the first client (the "speaker") will have one minute to talk about the topic while the second client (the "listener") listens.
3. During the first round, the listener is to use all the *ineffectual* attending behaviors he or she can think of while the spouse is talking. For example, shifting around in the chair, looking around the room, interrupting the speaker, or getting up and doing something else while partially listening. Although this portion of the exercise can be fun, at least for the listener, encourage him or her *not* to ham up the performance too much, but to be as realistic as possible.
4. Debrief both the listener's and the speaker's feelings about the exercise. Inquire with both partners how this might reflect everyday conversations they have with each other or with friends and family.
5. Next, have the clients reverse roles. The client who was the

speaker first is now the listener (who uses nonattending behaviors) and the client who was the listener first is now the speaker.
6. Again, debrief reactions to the role play.

Round 2

1. Ask one of the clients to be the speaker and talk about the same topic (or a more personal one) while the other client is the listener, this time practicing *effective* attending skills (i.e., eye contact, appropriate body posture) and reflective listening skills (i.e., paraphrasing and reflecting feelings).
2. Debrief reactions and again inquire of the couple how this type of communication is similar or dissimilar to their daily conversations with each other, family, and friends.
3. Have clients switch roles again and have the first speaker now practice effective attending and reflective listening skills.
4. Discuss clients' feelings and reactions to the different types of listening. Inquire how these different modes of listening and attending to each other could make a difference in their relationship. Also, inquire how learning these various skills could make a difference in their maintenance of sobriety.

Exercise

Have clients consciously practice these attending skills at home with each other. The therapist can then check in with clients every few sessions to determine whether they are indeed implementing these skills and how the new skills are working for them.

Case Illustration: Communication Skills

Mike and Beth indicated early on in treatment that communication was a problem for both of them in their first marriages and still is an area that they need to work on in their relationship. Beth complains that whenever she tries to talk to Mike about a serious topic, he begins joking around and trying to "lighten things up." Mike, on the other hand, complains that Beth repeats herself over and over and he has a difficult time listening to her. After the therapist introduces the Communication Skills exercises, Mike and Beth are able to identify a number of problems that contribute to their difficulties in communicating with each other. Mike realizes that when he attempts to "lighten things up," it is often because Beth wants to talk to him about something when he is distracted or tired. Beth realizes that she repeats herself because she does not feel like Mike is listening to her or truly hearing what she has to say.

The couple agree to make some changes. Mike agrees to tell Beth that he is tired or distracted if she tries to talk to him when he is unavailable, and to suggest a later time when they can talk. Beth agrees to tell Mike when she is not feeling heard, and to ask him if there is a better time to talk. Another skill that is particularly helpful for the couple is the "reflective listening" where Mike tells Beth what he hears her saying (paraphrasing) after she speaks, rather than being silent or giving her advice. Beth reports that when Mike actively listens, she does not feel the need to repeat herself over and over. Both partners state that this type of communication is awkward at first, especially when they use the "formula" they were taught in therapy. However, they also state that the more often they use these skills, the less likely they are to get into arguments and the more comfortable and relaxed they feel in communicating with each other.

COMMUNICATION SKILLS: LEVEL III

The third level of communication skills training introduces the technique of "giving and receiving feedback." This skill is a particularly important one for strengthening the therapeutic relationship, as well as enhancing the couple relationship. Typically, alcoholics are fairly sensitive to negative feedback, and fairly discounting of positive feedback. Thus, providing them with the structure and skills both to give and to receive feedback can be advantageous.

Skill 1: Giving and Receiving Feedback

As in any cognitive-behavioral therapy approach, a collaborative relationship between client and therapist is essential in order to enhance clients' motivation, to actively engage them in treatment, and to strengthen the therapeutic alliance. When clients feel that they are actively contributing to the therapy process, compliance is more likely. Because this treatment program involves a number of in-session activities, as well as out-of-session exercises, it is essential that the clients are active participants. Thus, it is important for the therapist both to give feedback to the clients as well as to receive feedback from them throughout therapy. In doing so, the therapist will be modelling another important communication technique and can use this as an opportunity to teach specific skills.

Rationale

Giving feedback to the clients regarding their behavior provides an opportunity to correct or modify any misconstructions made by the therapist. Beck et al. (1979) suggest that the therapist frequently give the client a "capsule summary" of the content and process going on during the session, so as to assure that they are on the same track (pp. 83–84).

Receiving feedback from the clients is essential in determining the level of understanding they have achieved throughout the program. Additionally, receiving feedback from the clients is important for exploring their perceptions and feelings about each session, about the exercises, and about the relationship with the therapist. All of these factors will affect the clients' participation and compliance with treatment; thus, it is vital to address any misunderstandings, resentments, or resistances as soon as possible. Feedback enables the therapist to adjust the therapeutic techniques and goals to fit the clients' levels of understanding and abilities.

1. Asking for feedback from, and giving feedback to, a client are important communication skills to model. Often, the alcoholic client has ineffective communication skills and will allow misunderstandings and assumptions to occur without knowing how to intervene. In research by Cummings et al. (1980), findings indicate that 16% of the relapses (in a population of 311 subjects, with varying addictive behaviors) were due to interpersonal conflict. Thus, modeling effective communication skills to clients is an important relapse prevention strategy.

2. The couple's relationship has been altered by the alcoholic's drinking as well, and it is likely that their communication has deteriorated. Giving and receiving feedback with the therapist may give the clients more confidence in utilizing this skill with each other. Examples are given throughout this section that explore how clients can apply giving and receiving feedback in their relationship.

Procedure

Step 1. An important part of the cognitive-behavioral collaborative model is to elicit evaluative feedback from clients. Clients are asked to discuss the usefulness of the interventions and the likelihood of implementing these interventions in daily living; for example, at the beginning of the session, the therapist may ask the clients in what way the suggested out-of-session exercises were helpful. Or, at the end of the session the therapist may ask what the clients learned during the session that will be useful, and specifically how they will use what they learned.

Step 2. Periodically, the therapist may also ask about the therapy in general. For example, the therapist might ask, "How is being in couple therapy helping you change your alcoholic behavior and thinking?" or, "In what ways have you made progress thus far and what other areas need to be addressed?"

Step 3. The therapist might also ask partners to identify the positive and negative changes they have noticed in each other since the beginning of the program. It is sometimes preferable, for example, when clients cannot readily answer these questions in the session, to assign an at-home exercise in which clients list behaviors they have improved and behaviors that still need improvement. Lists can then be discussed during the following session.

Step 4. Feedback may also be requested when the therapist needs input from clients on how well they understood a concept or an explanation of out-of-session exercises. It may be helpful to clients if the therapist elicits feedback regarding the clarity and understanding of each new concept or assignment presented.

Giving Feedback

When one person gives another feedback, the results can be positive or negative, and can hinder or further the relationship, depending on a variety of variables. One of the most important of these variables is the manner in which the feedback is delivered. Clients will increase the probability that feedback will enhance, rather than hinder, their relationship if they use the following guidelines.

Step 1. *Choose an appropriate time and place to give feedback.* Feedback should be given when the receiver is ready to hear it. Feedback is less useful when the receiver is overwhelmed by emotion. Further, there should be an appropriate amount of privacy—not in front of the children, at a party, and so forth. While keeping this in mind, it is also important to realize that the more immediate the feedback, the better. In therapy, the therapist and clients may decide ahead of time when to discuss feedback regarding previous sessions. For example, the therapist and clients may agree that each session will begin with a review and evaluation of the previous session. This plan allows for both immediacy and preparation (i.e., clients know ahead of time that they will be expected both to give and to receive feedback).

Step 2. *Feedback should be delivered in such a way as to minimize defensiveness and increase the probability that the receiver will be able to hear the information.* Using "I" messages can be very helpful because the person giving the feedback acknowledges that the feedback is simply his or her own opinion, not an undisputable fact. In addition to the "I" message, giving specifics regarding behavior and reasons for the feedback can be helpful. The formula that clients may use, which is introduced earlier in the Communication Skills: Level I component, is stated below.

Note that an addition to the formula is presented here. The last part of the formula adds a "specific request" to be made by the person giving the feedback. Often feedback is given back and forth and takes on the form of "complaining." Giving a specific request or suggestion gives the person receiving the feedback an opportunity to hear how he or she might change the behavior that is problematic for the person giving the feedback. The formula and an example follow:

"I feel _____ [emotion] when you _____ [behavior] because _____ [reason]. I request _____ [specific request]."

Example. During a therapy session a client tells his girlfriend that she's been "making him feel annoyed because she never comes home when she says she's going to." Her response is to explode at her partner because she "always comes home on time and he is just trying to control her." After exploring this comment with the couple, it becomes clear that on Wednesday nights when the girlfriend goes to an AA meeting, she often spends time socializing with friends and comes home later than she says she will be home. The partner worries that his girlfriend is out drinking. The therapist comments on the partner's feedback, including how he blames the girlfriend as opposed to taking responsibility for his feelings, as well as his use of the word "never," which often creates immediate defensiveness. After helping the partner formulate a message where he takes responsibility, gives specific feedback, and makes a request of his girlfriend, he is able to communicate the following message, "I feel annoyed when you say you will be home at 10 P.M. on Wednesday nights and you come home between 11 P.M. and 12 P.M. I am worried because I think you might be drinking and I get scared. I would like it if you called me if you were going to be later than 10:30 so I don't worry." The girlfriend then gets a chance to respond to the feedback and negotiate the request.

Step 3. *In giving feedback one should avoid name calling, labels, and judgmental words.* It is not helpful to hear, "You're neurotic, stupid, codependent, obsessed, trying to get back at your mother." Rather, focusing on the person's behavior that is in question will decrease defensiveness and be more useful. For example, when calling someone "codependent," it is difficult to know what that means or how it is a problem. A more effective way of giving someone feedback, rather than labeling, is to say, "when you tell your friends that your husband is at home sick, rather than he is in bed because he drank too much last night, this behavior may enable your husband to avoid facing the consequences of his drinking." This latter statement avoids any labeling and is descriptive rather than judgmental.

Step 4. *Feedback should be descriptive rather than interpretive:* that is, the giver should not guess at the receiver's motives or intentions. For example, it is *not* helpful to say, "The reason you bought that bottle of bourbon was to get even with me for yelling at your mother." Rather, the giver can express feedback, using an "I" message and ask what the motive or intention might have been for the other person's behavior. For example, "I was concerned when you bought the bourbon, and I'm wondering if it has anything to do with my argument with your mother." The therapist can role model this point when giving clients feedback during sessions. Rather than making interpretations, the therapist can be also be descriptive and inquire about motivations. For example, when a client does not complete at-home exercises three sessions in a row, the therapist might say, "I've noticed that in the beginning of treatment you consistently completed the at-home exercises we agreed on. For the past 3 weeks, however, you have not completed the assignments, and I'm wondering what might be going on?" This is very different than an interpretation about why the client might not be completing assignments, as in, "It appears that for the past 3 weeks you might be less invested in treatment because you've not been completing the assignment."

Step 5. *Feedback should be limited to one aspect of behavior,* not, for example, "I'm upset because you were 2 hours late and you forgot to get gas and you didn't feed the dog and you lost my flashlight." A comment such as, "I'm upset because I worked hard to have dinner ready at 6:00 and you didn't get home until 8:00," may be more easily heard by the receiver. In therapy, the therapist might help the clients practice this aspect of giving feedback by asking for *one* thing about the previous session that was helpful, especially when the clients respond, "Oh, everything was really great."

Step 6. *Feedback should refer only to something that can be modified.* There is no point in giving feedback to someone about something he or she can do nothing about (e.g., "Over and over again you prove that you really aren't very smart," or, "Your ears really do stick out"). A good rule of thumb is that feedback should be directed at a person's *behavior,* rather than personal attributes.

Receiving Feedback

Most people become defensive when anyone takes exception to their behavior. Clients should be taught how to receive as well as to give feedback. The following steps may be helpful in teaching clients to respond to negative feedback about themselves by listening carefully to what the partner (or someone else) is saying and by reflecting content and feelings of the message. Often people begin "rehearsing" their response to the feedback and miss a good portion of the message. The following strategies might be helpful.

Step 1. Review with clients the following typical reactions to receiving negative feedback and ask for examples of each:

1. *Denial.* The person denies that the behavior occurred ("I didn't do it") or denies the giver's emotions ("You shouldn't feel that way. You're overreacting").
2. *Rationalization.* The person excuses him- or herself in any number of ways, for example, "What I meant was . . . ," or, "I was trying to . . . ," or, "I did it that way because. . . ."
3. *Attack.* The receiver turns on the giver of feedback. "Oh yeah? What about the time you crashed the Volvo . . . ?"

Step 2. *Choose an appropriate time and setting* to receive the feedback. The receiver has every right to choose the time and place for feedback, just as the giver of the feedback does.

Step 3. Have the client's first goal be to *repeat the feedback back to the speaker, without any edits, responses, or interpretations.* For example, in a scenario where the therapist has given a client feedback about her enabling behavior, the therapist can ask the client first to repeat back to the therapist what she heard the therapist saying. If the client "edits" the feedback, the therapist can correct the client and again ask her to repeat exactly what was said.

Step 4. Once the feedback has been repeated and thus received, encourage the receiver to *take a moment to "check in,"* and encourage them to take a moment to breathe and notice how they are feeling.

Step 5. Respond to the feedback using the "I" message formula, modified as follows:

"When you said _____ [accurate statement, without edits] I felt _____ [emotion] because _____ [reason]."

"I think the part of the feedback that is accurate is _____ ."

"I think the part of the feedback that is inaccurate is _____ ."

This formula gives the client a chance to practice looking at what part of the feedback might be accurate, rather than immediately discounting it because part of it doesn't fit.

Step 6. Receiver gets a chance to respond to the specific request and negotiate, if appropriate (see Step 2 in the Giving Feedback section above).

Step 7. Repeat this process between giver and receiver of feedback until communication is clear.

Exercises

1. Have clients practice giving each other feedback on nonthreatening issues and report back the interchange. As clients get more comfortable giving and receiving feedback, they may practice with more personal issues.

2. Have clients note times in the week when someone gave them feedback, or they gave someone else feedback. In addition, have clients note what aspect of the experience went well and where they may have had difficulty. Bring notes to session for review and problem solving.

3. With respect to giving and receiving feedback with the therapist, if clients have difficulty verbalizing how they feel about the session or their relationship with the therapist, have them write it down between each session. Having written it down, the clients may find it easier to begin by reading their reactions to the therapist. The long-term goal, of course, is to have the clients spontaneously share their feedback about the session and their relationship with the therapist. This can also be used with couples who are having a difficult time giving and/or receiving feedback with each other.

Recommendations

In the 20-session model, communication skills are primarily introduced in the Early Treatment Phase (Sessions 4–7) and reinforced throughout the remainder of treatment. We recommend communication skills training in the Early Treatment Phase because the training can give the couple immediate tools to implement both insession and out of session. In our program, clients often report that the benefits from implementing these basic communication skills were noticeable in their relationships right away, which gave them hope and increased their motivation for working on problems with each other. These skills can, however, be implemented at any time during treatment, as deemed appropriate by the therapist.

CHAPTER 6

Phase III:
Middle Treatment

Overview

Self-Monitoring: Level II
- Drinking Chain II and Target Behavior Chart II

Cognitive Coping Skills: Alternative Thoughts
Behavioral Coping Skills
Drink/Target Behavior Refusal Skills
Termination of Acute Phase of Treatment

Materials Needed:
- Drinking Chain II and Target Behavior Chart II (Forms 6 and 7)
- Drink/Target Behavior Refusal Rules (Forms 8a, 8b)
- Exercise Records (Form 3)
- Pencils and Clipboards

Recommended number of sessions: 5

Goals: 1. Teach more complex self-monitoring skills.
2. Explore coping skills and resources.
3. Teach drink/target behavior refusal skills.
4. Set the stage for the Relapse Prevention Phase of treatment.

The Middle Treatment Phase outlined in Chapter 6 is designed to build upon the skills introduced in the Early Treatment Phase and to prepare clients for the Relapse Prevention Phase by teaching them more advanced coping strategies, including drink/target behavior refusal. This chapter begins with Level II of Self-Monitoring, which sets the stage for clients to learn cognitive and behavioral coping skills to deal with dysfunctional thoughts and feelings. Following the introduction of these various cognitive and behavioral coping skills, suggestions for terminating the acute phase of treatment are offered and preparation for relapse prevention is initiated. The Middle Phase of Treatment is an ideal time to either continue with Level I and II of the Communication Skills and/or introduce the Level III skills.

Note that in order to move to the Relapse Prevention Phase, the clients must be abstinent from alcohol and the target behavior. If clients are having difficulty with this goal, it may be necessary to slow down or readjust the treatment plan.

SELF-MONITORING: LEVEL II

The self-monitoring introduced in the Early Treatment Phase is taken to a new level as therapy progresses. As you will recall, the purpose of self-monitoring in the Early Treatment Phase is to help clients begin to understand the types of stimuli that trigger them to drink and engage in the target behavior. In this second level of exploring triggers, clients are introduced to new charts—Drinking Chain II and Target Behavior Chart II (Forms 6 and 7). These new charts have two new columns, which help the clients break down the identified triggers into thoughts and feelings. As the clients are more specific about their triggers to drink or engage in a target behavior, they will learn more effective, more appropriate coping strategies. In particular, as clients become more aware of their automatic thoughts and feelings, they will learn both cognitive and behavioral coping strategies to respond effectively to such triggers.

Rationale

The Drinking Chain I and Target Behavior Chart I were presented to the clients in order to introduce the idea that there is a relationship between environmental stimuli (people, places, and events) and the clients' urge to drink or engage in a target behavior. The Drinking Chain II and Target Behavior Chart II are now introduced to refine this concept further and to teach the clients that it is actually their interpretation of the stimuli that results in the urge to drink or engage in the behavior. They are also taught that feelings are often the mediating factor between these interpretations, or thoughts, and the behavior.

1. Alcoholics are known to have particular cognitive distortions and rationalizations that result in drinking. Common examples of these dysfunctional cognitions are, "I can have just one beer and then go home,"

and, "I've already blown it once this week, I might as well drink again." Marlatt and Gordon (1985), in their book *Relapse Prevention: Maintenance Strategies in the Treatment of Addictive Behaviors,* cite the most frequently observed distortions: overgeneralization, selective abstraction, and catastrophizing. Often, these distortions and rationalizations are automatic thoughts of which the alcoholic is unaware. Thus, it is critical that the alcoholic recognize these thoughts and learn strategies for dealing with them. The rationale is that the more functional and realistic the thoughts and interpretations are, the more likely that the alcoholic's behavior will be consistent with his or her goal to remain abstinent.

2. The Drinking Chain II and Target Behavior Chart II, as with the previous charts, are ways to help clients self-monitor daily thoughts and feelings and recognize those thoughts and feelings that reinforce abstinence and those that do not. The charts are adapted from Beck and colleagues' (1979, p. 288) "Daily Record of Dysfunctional Thoughts" and are the vehicle from which to identify patterns, teach the clients about countering dysfunctional thoughts, and explore alternative behavioral coping strategies.

Procedure

The assumption in cognitive therapy about the relationship between thoughts and feelings is deceptively simple. Often clients say that they understand the idea, but later it becomes clear that they have only limited comprehension of this concept. It is important to take this portion of the therapy slowly. Explain the concept carefully with the use of frequent examples to be certain that the clients do, in fact, grasp the idea that thoughts create feelings.

Step 1. Begin by presenting the idea that it is important to understand one's automatic thoughts and feelings in order to be more effective in intervening with a situation when one is tempted to use alcohol or another drug, or to engage in the target behavior. Then discuss the concept that one's thoughts create feelings; situations or events do not create feelings. Repeat this concept in different words, for example, "Many people believe that feelings, such as joy, sadness,or anger are caused by other people's behavior or by other outside influences. In reality, our feelings are caused by the thoughts and beliefs we have *about* an event or *about* someone else's behavior."

Step 2. Next, provide several examples showing how the same situation can trigger different feelings, depending on the person's thoughts. It is easier for clients to learn the concepts if you chart the

examples on a blackboard as you tell the story. Three specific examples
follow; however, it might be necessary to create new examples that are
more relevant to the clients' ages and life situations. Be careful not to
use examples that relate to alcohol, to a marital problem, or to any other
topic that might engage strong feelings in the clients that would cause
them to pay more attention to the examples than to the concepts that
you are attempting to teach.

1. Begin by listing the following categories on a blackboard or piece
of paper:

SITUATION   THOUGHTS   FEELINGS

Begin the narrative as follows: Eddie graduates from high school and
decides, with his parents' reluctant permission, to drive across the country
with a friend. Eddie agrees to telephone or write home at least once a
week. The first 2 weeks, the parents get letters from Eddie, then there is
silence. Four weeks have passed without a word, and the parents become
increasingly worried. Then a letter arrives from Eddie. (Write "Letter from
Eddie" on the blackboard under SITUATION.)
    Eddie's mother cries tears of joy, and his father's reaction is anger.
(On the blackboard under FEELINGS write "Mother: Joy," and "Father:
Anger.")
    Because the parents are both reading the same letter, the letter itself
cannot be responsible for their dissimilar feelings. Although each parent
reads the same letter, the thoughts of each are very different. When Eddie's
mother reads the letter, she thinks, "Thank God he's alive." As a result,
she feels joy. When Eddie's father reads the letter he thinks, "How dare
he worry us by not writing earlier." As a result, he feels anger. (On the
blackboard under THOUGHTS add "Thank God he's alive" and "How
dare he worry us?"):

SITUATION	THOUGHTS	FEELINGS
Letter from	Thank God he's alive.	Mother: Joy
Eddie	How dare he worry us?	Father: Anger

Thus, the letter itself did not cause the emotions, it was the thoughts
the parents had *about* the letter that were responsible for their feelings.

2. Provide another example, charting it on the blackboard in the
same manner. This time elicit input from the clients. An example may be
as follows: Mr. Smith's physician tells him that his blood pressure is still
high, but did not increase in the last month.
    What thoughts might cause Mr. Smith to feel depressed about this

news? Try to elicit appropriate thoughts from clients and write them on the board. If clients fail to name suitable thoughts, supply them yourself. For example, if Mr. Smith thinks, "It's no better, I'm never going to get better," he will cause himself to feel depressed or anxious.

Given the same situation, what thoughts might cause Mr. Smith to feel relieved? Again, attempt to elicit appropriate thought statements from the clients and, if they have difficulty coming up with thoughts, help them. Again, summarize: In response to the same situation, if Mr. Smith thinks, "At least it's no worse; maybe it's on the mend," instead of feeling depressed he will feel positive, perhaps relieved, or even hopeful.

SITUATION	THOUGHTS	FEELINGS
Blood pressure	I'll never get better.	Depressed
still high	At least it's not worse.	Relieved

3. The third example should require clients to fill in most of the blanks. The first week of her freshman year at university, Sally meets Ralph, who asks her to a party Saturday night. Saturday night arrives, but Ralph doesn't. Sally is stood up. What might Sally feel? List on the blackboard three to five emotions that the clients name. If clients list a number of words that mean the same thing, choose just one for the blackboard, for example, instead of "angry, riled, mad, irked, pissed off," simply write "Angry." Again, if necessary, add feelings that they might have missed.

Ask the clients what thoughts Sally must have in order to produce each of these feelings? Take each feeling in turn, elicit from the clients thoughts that would be likely to trigger each of the listed feelings.

SITUATION	THOUGHTS	FEELINGS
Stood up	I thought he liked me.	Hurt
	He's got his nerve.	Angry
	I was looking forward to seeing him.	Disappointed
		Relieved
	I didn't really like him very much.	Scared
	Nobody wants to go out with me.	

4. The final examples should be from the clients' own lives. Again, put the headings on the blackboard and work first with one client, then with the other. Have each of them identify an incident in the past week in which they felt "upset." Ask the clients to describe the situation, and in two or three words write it on the board. Then have the clients identify the feelings that they experienced in that situation. Ask the clients to identify the thoughts that led to the feelings.

Step 3. When you are sure that the clients understand this concept, hand out copies of the Drinking Chain II and the Target Behavior Chart II (Forms 6 and 7). Explain that the same concept of "thoughts create feelings" applies when one is tempted to use alcohol or engage in a target behavior. Go over the example on the forms and have clients fill in at least one recent incident in which they had a thought to use alcohol or engage in the target behavior. On the back side of the charts is an extensive list of feelings for clients who have difficulty identifying emotions. It is often helpful to take time to help clients distinguish between thoughts and emotions and help them learn ways to identify emotions. Many alcoholics, after years of drinking, have become numb to emotions and "go blank" when asked how they are feeling, or they tell you how they are thinking instead. The list of feeling words is often very useful with this type of client. Most importantly, be patient. Usually, emotions begin to surface slowly and it may take time before a client is able to identify his or her feelings accurately. In some cases, however, emotions surface rather quickly once an alcoholic quits drinking and this experience can be overwhelming for the client who has numbed him- or herself for years. In either case, it is critical to help clients identify their feelings and cope with them in adaptive, healthy ways, rather than drinking.

Step 4. For clients who have difficulty accessing their automatic thoughts, you may consider having them start by filling in the feelings column and working backwards. We have found that some clients can access their feelings more readily and can only access the thoughts once they have figured out what they were feeling. Over time, clients are usually able to notice and "capture" the automatic thoughts more easily.

Reviewing Charts

It is recommended that the clients complete the charts daily as with the original self-monitoring charts. If clients are continuing to have numerous triggers to drink or engage in the target behavior daily, you may want to have them enter at least the most salient craving each day because the new charts are more time consuming.

Step 1. In the session following the introduction of the new charts, it is important to reinforce any attempts to complete these charts. Clients may have difficulty at first, usually in that they are not specific or detailed enough in their entries. As the sessions progress, clients usually become more efficient at completing the new columns.

Step 2. Review charts as you have in previous sessions. However, now that the trigger column is broken down into two new columns, "thoughts" and "feelings," you will want to spend more time exploring these entries. Along with the clients, begin to get a picture of the thoughts that reinforce abstinence, leading to a "No" in the results column, and those that reinforce drinking, leading to a "Yes." For example (refer to Example 1, Form 6), when the client thought, "I haven't had a drink in 3 weeks, one glass won't hurt," he ended up drinking. He felt "deprived and left out" at first and then "pleased" once he started drinking. Obviously these thoughts are dangerous for the client and lead to drinking. In the second example, the client thinks to himself, "I usually drink beer when I watch the game, but I am trying to quit," and this thought results in abstinence.

Step 3. Review the results and alternatives column. What happened as a result of the client's decision? Sometimes the client feels better because he or she did not drink, and sometimes the client feels worse (e.g., more angry or more depressed). This will give you an idea of what type of coping strategies will be needed. For example, the client may need more coping skills to deal with difficult emotions and high-risk situations, or the client may need help in coming up with alternative thoughts that are more uplifting and encouraging.

Step 4. Spend time helping clients come up with alternative coping strategies, both cognitive and behavioral, that are appropriate for each entry on their charts. In the following section, we review these types of interventions.

Exercises

1. Have clients complete the new charts, Drinking Chain II and Target Behavior Chart II, daily.
2. Review the charts in each session throughout the Middle Treatment Phase, with an emphasis on learning new cognitive and behavioral strategies to cope with triggers.

COGNITIVE COPING SKILLS: ALTERNATIVE THOUGHTS

Once the clients have begun to use the Drinking Chain II and Target Behavior Chart II regularly, and they are able to identify specific coping deficiencies, it is important to introduce therapeutic interventions that address these deficiencies. Two approaches are offered in this chapter: (1) a cognitive therapy approach whereby clients are taught how to challenge their automatic thoughts and counter them with rational, abstinence oriented thoughts (vs. drinking-oriented thoughts) and (2) a behavior therapy approach whereby clients are taught how to enhance their sobriety by changing behaviors when confronted with high-risk situations from an automatic drinking response to a more functional behavioral response (e.g., calling a friend, going for a walk, etc.). This section addresses the cognitive techniques and the following section addresses the behavioral techniques. The cognitive techniques section focuses on the alcoholic behavior; however, the techniques may easily be applied to most target behaviors.

Rationale

As presented in the previous section, alcoholics have well-known cognitive distortions that serve to reinforce drinking behavior. *Catastrophizing* an event, for example, will often give the alcoholic an "excuse" to drink. Another example that may lead the alcoholic to drink is *overgeneralizing* a problem and believing that it will "always" be present and will "never" get better. *Minimizing* the seriousness of the alcohol problem is another common distortion that serves to reinforce drinking and interfere with treatment. There are quite a number of other types of cognitive distortions, including all-or-nothing thinking, mind reading, selective abstraction, jumping to conclusions, labeling, and "should" statements that create negative affect, thus triggering the alcoholic to drink.

1. Although there are many cognitive restructuring techniques to deal with distortions and irrational thinking, this book focuses on the "countering" technique. Countering helps clients argue against the irrational, maladaptive thoughts that reinforce drinking, and also challenges clients to come up with rational, adaptive thoughts that reinforce abstinence.

2. McMullin (1986), in *Handbook of Cognitive Therapy Techniques*, states that there is a single theory underlying the cognitive restructuring technique of countering. This theory asserts that "when a client argues against an irrational thought, and does so repeatedly, the irrational thought becomes progressively weaker" (p. 3). The process does not happen magically, but occurs over time as a result of the counterthought eliciting affect that reduces the negative emotion or "removes the stimulus triggering this emotion" (p. 3). Thus, countering irrational thoughts can be a powerful tool for clients to learn, although it is one that must be practiced diligently.

3. Kadden et al. (1989), in their research manual for working with alcohol-abusing and alcohol-dependent individuals, contend that the automatic negative thoughts that alcoholic individuals often experience

lead to depression. The depression then leads to increased negative thoughts and increased likelihood that the alcoholic will believe these thoughts. This process of negative thinking and depression can become a significant trigger for drinking. Thus, the alcoholic must learn active ways to become aware of these automatic thoughts and begin to challenge them.

Procedure

As Kadden and colleagues (1989) point out, the first step in dealing with automatic, negative thoughts is to become more aware of their existence. Given that these thoughts are automatic, the alcoholic is often unaware of them. What the alcoholic is aware of usually is the negative emotions that result from this type of thinking (e.g., sadness, anger, frustration). Some alcoholics are unaware of both the automatic thoughts and the resulting emotions. When working with this type of client, the therapist might hear from him or her, "I don't know what happened. I was driving home and the next thing I knew, I was at the bar drinking." For this reason, the Drinking Chain II and Target Behavior Chart II are designed to have clients list thoughts, feelings, and results to the best of their ability. It will become clear to the therapist rather quickly where the focus needs to be initially; that is, whether the client need help "capturing" the automatic thoughts and/or identifying emotions that are triggers to the drinking/target behavior. The following procedure outlines the basic steps to teaching the countering technique. The therapist may choose to incorporate additional cognitive restructuring techniques at this point, or later in treatment when clients master the basic countering.

Step 1. Explain the basic concepts underlying cognitive therapy and, in particular, countering. It is often helpful to frame this technique as a coping strategy that the client *always* has available; that is, he or she does not need to rely on anyone or anything else to apply this coping strategy. Once clients master this technique and practice it regularly, countering can be a beneficial, immediate coping strategy to count on in many high-risk situations.

Step 2. There are a number of ways to begin teaching the countering technique. One possibility is to share with clients a list of cognitive distortions. Burns (1989), for instance, has a useful chart called the "Checklist of Cognitive Distortions" (p. 96). A list may help the clients begin to notice their thinking patterns. Another possibility is to have the clients list as many thoughts as they can that have triggered them to drink in thee past. It is often helpful for clients to think of past drinking episodes rather than trying to capture the current thoughts. Examples of these types of thoughts include, "I can have just one," "I will quit tomorrow," "I am so stressed," "I have been abstinent for 3 weeks, I have proven that I can quit," and "No one believes I can really quit so I might as well drink." A third option is to start with using the thoughts that clients have been recording on the Drinking Chain II or Target Behavior Chart II.

Step 3. Once clients are able to identify some automatic thoughts, the therapist may ask what emotions are elicited by these thoughts. The Drinking Chain II and Target Behavior Chart II can be useful in this exploration. For example, if a client thinks, "No one believes I can really quit, so I might as well drink," explore what emotions this thought elicits. Perhaps this thought leads the client to feel "hopeless," "alone," or "sad."

It can also be helpful to have the clients rate the intensity of the emotion. The purpose of this strategy is to teach clients how to counter their thoughts, and to measure the effectiveness of the countered thought. An effective countered thought is determined by the degree to which it decreases negative emotion and increases positive emotion.

Step 4. The clients are now ready to learn how to challenge their automatic thoughts. The first step is to question the rationality or the truthfulness of the thought, as well as to question whether the thought is reinforcing of abstinent behavior or drinking behavior.

1. What is the evidence for this thought?
2. What is another way to look at this event?
3. Am I distorting [review checklist]?
4. Would my wife [husband, therapist, or friend, who is supportive of my abstinence] agree with this thought? Why not?
5. Am I making some *assumptions* here?
6. If I believe this thought, what will most likely happen?
7. Does this thought reinforce my abstinence or my drinking?

It may also be helpful to review the event to which the client is responding (recorded on the Drinking Chain II and Target Behavior Chart II in the situation column) and to explore alternative *interpretations* of this event. The point of challenging the automatic thoughts is to have the clients understand that these are just thoughts and that years of repeating them and believing them have made these thoughts appear as facts to be acted on.

Step 5. Once clients have begun to challenge their automatic thoughts, they are ready to counter them, that is, consciously to formulate new thoughts that are rational, honest, and adaptive to sobriety. The therapist may begin by having clients list as many counterthoughts as possible. Usually clients can come up with about one or two initially. The next step might be to have the client ask his or her partner for ideas of counterthoughts and write down those that make the most sense. The therapist may then add some additional counterthoughts to the list. For example:

Negative thought

+ "No one believes I can really quit, so I might as well drink."

Counterthoughts

+ "Actually, it is not true that no one believes in me, my wife does because she is in therapy with me."
+ "I quit once before for 5 years, so I really can quit if I am committed."
+ "I could drink right now, but if I do, I will keep drinking until I pass out and then I will really have trouble."

Step 6. Another useful strategy is to have the client "answer" the negative thought and then formulate a counterthought. Using the example above, the client might answer the negative thought with, "It is true that some people do not believe I can quit because, in truth, I have said I was going to quit many times in the past." Then, the counter could be, "However, I did quit once before for 5 years. I am now in a treatment program for alcoholism and I've never tried that before." The purpose of "answering" the negative thought is to reinforce the idea that the client is not to "ignore" the negative thought but, rather, to acknowledge the thought and counter it with a rational, adaptive thought. While initially learning this technique, clients will often hear that they are to "ignore" their irrational thoughts and "think positively." Ignoring usually does not work for long, if at all, and while thinking positively may be a helpful strategy for some, the countering technique is more powerful and enduring.

Step 7. Some basic guidelines for formulating counterthoughts are as follows:

1. The counterthought needs to be believable.
2. The client should come up with a thought that is realistic—not just a "positive affirmation"—and it should be specific.
3. The counterthought should decrease the negative affect the original thought elicited.
4. Clients should be taught that practice is the key to having this technique work in daily living.

Step 8. Have clients note how they feel about the new counter-thought; that is, did the emotion elicited from the original negative thought lessen? If so, the counterthought is an effective one; if not, then other counterthoughts should be explored.

Step 9. Have clients go over entries on the Drinking Chain II and Target Behavior Chart II and counter all of the thoughts in the thoughts column. Notice the effect on their feelings, and hypothesize about the likely result if this new strategy had been employed.

Step 10. Clients can also role play different scenarios with each other (see section below on Drink/Target Behavior Refusal Skills), practice how to challenge the thoughts, and then practice how to counter them with rational, abstinence-oriented thoughts.

Exercises

1. Have clients practice countering negative thoughts at home. Writing down the negative thoughts and the counterthoughts can be particularly helpful in the beginning.

2. Have clients challenge each other when they hear cognitive distortions from each other. It may be necessary to help clients find ways to challenge each other in a supportive manner.

3. Have clients ask for feedback from their partners when trying to formulate counterthoughts. This may help the clients formulate more effective thoughts, as well as reinforce collaboration in working through problems.

4. Continue to elicit counterthoughts from clients during each session in which the Drinking Chain II and Target Behavior Chart II are utilized.

BEHAVIORAL COPING SKILLS

This section offers three behavioral interventions to use in couple therapy to help therapists address coping deficiencies. The interventions are (1) assessment of the clients' coping resources, (2) exploration of ways the clients can enhance their resource base, and (3) skills training.

Rationale

Research on relapse episodes confirms what many practitioners already know; that is, the coping skills available to many alcoholics are inadequate

(Marlatt & Gordon, 1985). Addressing these inadequacies is a critical component of any treatment and relapse prevention plan.

1. Assessment of the clients' coping resources is the first step in addressing their needs. Coping resources refer to beliefs and skills a person may draw upon to deal with the demands of everyday living, as well as the demands of stressful events. These resources may include material resources, health and energy, spiritual beliefs, social support, social skills, and problem-solving skills (Lazarus & Folkman, 1984). Exploring availability of these resources to the clients, as well as the clients' ability to access these resources, is important.

2. As treatment progresses, reviewing the clients' Drinking Chains I and II and Target Behavior Charts I and II will give the therapist information about the relationships between drinking or engaging in the target behavior, and deficiencies in coping resources. Clients often regard skills training, whether it be in social skills, communication skills, or problem-solving skills, as the most critical component of treatment. After drinking for many years, alcoholics often find themselves feeling embarrassed and incompetent when attempting many activities sober. For example, clients who have not interacted socially with others without drinking for many years may feel inadequate starting conversations with strangers when they are abstinent. In treatment, discussing, role playing, and rehearsing various social encounters or conflicts can be extremely helpful to clients and can decrease the chances of a relapse when they confront such situations.

Procedure

Step 1. One way to begin discussing alternative ways to cope with high-risk situations and emotions that are triggers to drink or engage in target behavior is to introduce the abbreviated Relapse Prevention Model by Marlatt and Gordon (1985; Appendix 4). The therapist can illustrate how coping plays a major role in the prevention of relapse and how important it is to have readily available coping strategies when confronted a difficult situation.

Step 2. Ask clients for examples from their past when they used strategies, other than drinking, to cope with a trigger to drink or engage in the target behavior, and discuss the consequences. Additionally, ask for examples of when the clients did *not* engage in effective strategies, and then discuss what the consequences were in this example. When you think the clients understand the concept of "coping" and the relationship between coping and relapse prevention, continue.

Step 3. The following are suggestions for exploring the clients' current strategies and resources and for discovering new ones.

1. Elicit from the couple a list of situations related to drinking that either typically cause them problems or might cause trouble once they are sober. The therapist should have handy a list of typical situations in order to be sure that all eventualities are considered. For example, situations at work, at home, with extended family, on vacation, at parties, with friends, or at sporting events.

2. Select one of these situations and have the clients walk through it until they can identify the point at which things first start to go wrong. What are their thoughts, their feelings, and their behavior at this point? How do they help or hinder each other? Especially, what do they do that makes the situation worse?

3. Using the situation they chose, have the couple identify alternative resources they could tap. These resources might include alternative thoughts, material resources, spiritual beliefs, social support, or problem-solving skills. Focus on how they can help each other, how they can use tactics such as distraction, self-talk, and so forth. Be sure to explain the importance of intervening early before the battle is lost, and be sure to include the partner in the effort to identify alternatives. Ask the partner to consider what he or she could have done differently to provide better support.

4. Similarly, have the clients make plans to "turn the tide" even later on in the scenario. Make the point that once headed down a particular road, it is not necessary to continue down it; that is, it is almost never too late to do something to change directions.

Step 4. Ask clients to make plans to reinforce each other for even partial success in coping with a difficult situation. For example, a partner might say to an alcoholic spouse, "I'm glad that you brought this up in therapy because you used to keep all these thoughts inside;" or, "I know this is difficult for you and it scares me when you drink, but I am proud of you for talking about it."

Step 5. As you go through each scenario with the clients, help them identify the strengths of their coping resources as well as the areas that need enhancing. It may be helpful if you actually write down the resources they come up with when going over each scenario. For example, a client's *strengths* might include having many close friends with whom to share feelings, having a supportive partner who is willing to be in treatment, and having good insurance or financial resources to cover costs of therapy and allow the patient to take a few weeks off work. *Areas to improve* might include coming up with alternative thoughts when offered a drink, developing stronger spiritual beliefs to strengthen hope and enhance sobriety, and increasing an exercise plan in order to feel healthier and have more energy.

Exercises

1. Ask clients to choose a potentially troublesome situation that is likely to occur during the upcoming week and to make detailed plans to cope with this situation using as many resources as possible. Have them report the following week, and at that time help them refine their coping techniques. Repeat this exercise as often as appropriate and check in with clients to determine how effectively they are able to integrate these new coping skills into their daily lives.

2. Make a general list of available coping resources, including supportive friends, activities, material goods, spiritual beliefs or affiliations, and so forth.

3. Make a list of all family and friends whom clients consider supportive and write down the ways they can be counted on in time of need (see Form 9 and Chapter 7 for further details on this suggested assignment).

4. Suggest the couple attend church (or other place of worship) once between sessions if they have been talking about going and keep putting it off, or go to an AA or Al-Anon meeting if they have never been (recommend that they try different meetings before deciding whether they like it or not). Also, if they used to attend AA and haven't been going because of a relapse, encourage them to go back.

5. List activities in which they could participate if they have an urge to drink or engage in the target behavior.

6. Have the couple discuss ways they could save money for enjoyable activities when they need an "escape" or "time-out" from their routines.

7. Throughout the remainder of the program, encourage clients to take risks to enhance their coping resources (e.g., making new friends, attending AA, sharing with friends and family their successes in treatment, taking up a new hobby, exercising).

Note. The following is an example of how coping skills training may be introduced to a couple in which the female partner is the alcoholic.

Case Illustration: Coping Skills

The alcoholic client, Sarah, was on a business trip to Europe recently and she relapsed after 3 weeks of abstinence. After careful analysis of the events leading up to the business trip, it becomes evident that Sarah was nervous about flying, remembered a story about a plane crash she heard on the radio the previous night, and thought that having "one drink" to calm herself wouldn't hurt. The client's husband, Mark, knew she was nervous about flying, worried about how Sarah would react when the stewardess offered her a drink, but said nothing to his wife, for fear she would get angry and defensive. He reports to the therapist that he just "hoped she would be strong enough to handle the situation."

While exploring alternative coping skills and resources, Sarah comes up with the following strategies. *Alternative thoughts* to counter the automatic thought about "having one drink to calm myself" include, "Yes, I could *start* with one drink to calm myself, but I've been sober for 3 weeks now and I want to maintain my sobriety," and, "I know if I have one drink that I will continue to drink throughout my trip and I am committed to staying sober" (this was her "Broken record" phrase, the concept of which is discussed below in Suggestions for the Design of the Role Play), and, "Yes, one drink would relax me, but five drinks, which is what I would probably have, would make me rude and obnoxious to the other passengers." *Material resources* she realizes are available and easily accessible include headsets for listening to music, a novel she had brought with her to read, and a relaxation tape that she had packed in her briefcase. *Social support* she could have engaged might have included the passenger beside her or the flight crew. (It would not be necessary for Sarah to reveal that she is an alcoholic if she is not comfortable doing so, but she could have discussed her nervousness, or her excitement about going to Europe.) Additionally, prior to the trip, Sarah could have shared her concerns with her husband or another friend, rather than keeping them to herself. Mark also realizes that he could have expressed his concern to Sarah by using the "I" messages they had practiced in therapy, or simply asking her how she was feeling about traveling.

After exploring these alternative coping resources, the therapist can pose the following situations to Sarah and Mark:

1. Sarah has had one drink and is considering having another; have her go through the same process outlined above of reviewing of cognitive and behavioral interventions and available resources. This will help Sarah realize that it is never too late to intervene with herself to "get back on track."

2. Sarah did not have the first drink offered her during take off, but then there is excessive turbulence and she begins to reconsider, especially when they offer free drinks. Again, have her identify appropriate interventions.

3. What might Mark have done differently in the original scenario and what he might have done if he were with Sarah on the plane and she started drinking?

DRINK/TARGET BEHAVIOR REFUSAL SKILLS

An important skill for alcoholic clients to learn in treatment is how to refuse a drink effectively. In this therapy approach, this skill is taught with the use of behavioral rehearsal, coaching, cognitive rehearsal, covert rehearsal, and videotaping. This skill is also applicable for most target behaviors from which the partner is abstaining and is a great way to involve the couple in actively supporting each other.

Rationale

It is important for the alcoholic to know how to say "no," how to stick to this decision, and how to prevent other people from hassling him or her. The same applies to the partner's abstention from a target behavior. Being able to say "no" assertively allows clients to direct their own lives, rather than permitting others to do so for them, and it allows the clients to build a sense of confidence in their ability to master drinking and target behavior problems. This skill can be applied in social situations when the client is offered a drink or asked to engage in the target behavior (e.g., eat a chocolate dessert when abstaining from sweets). The skill can also be used when the pressure is internal, that is, when the voice offering the drink is in the alcoholic's own head. For example, the familiar voice that says, "I'll just have one," or, "I'll just stop at the bar for a few minutes and order a soda."

1. Many alcoholics socialize with friends who are heavy drinkers, and drinking is often the primary activity in which they engage, or, at least, it accompanies their other activities. When they are learning to abstain from alcohol, many alcoholics are very concerned about having to give up their old friends and find a whole new set of friends with whom to socialize. This concern is valid and needs to be addressed. One way to address this issue is to teach the clients how to say "no" to alcohol in a way that creates as little defensiveness as possible and allows them to keep their old friends. The "broken record" is a refusal technique that is a very effective means of saying "no" without preaching or arguing (M. J. Smith, 1975).

2. In the study done by Cummings et al. (1980) that categorized relapse episodes among clients with a variety of addictive problems, the researchers found that approximately 20% of all these episodes were a result of "social pressure." This pressure was either direct, where the drinker is verbally persuaded to have a drink, or indirect, where the drinker was merely in the presence of other people who were drinking. Whether the pressure is direct or indirect, the alcoholic must learn to respond quickly when the temptation arises and to have a coping strategy

that is accessible in any situation that arises. Again, the "broken record" phrase is an ideal strategy because the alcoholic does not need to rely on others and does not need to leave the situation in order to prevent a relapse.

   3. Role playing of refusal situations gives the clients a chance to practice this skill and build some confidence in its effectiveness. Role playing is commonly employed in cognitive and and behavioral therapy (Beck et al., 1979; Wilson, 1989). Research has found that role playing is effective in helping alcoholics cope with problematic situations (Chaney, O'Leary, & Marlatt, 1978).

Procedure

The many techniques of role playing, or behavioral rehearsal, can be combined in a variety of ways to help the alcoholic and his or her partner learn to refuse a drink or targeted behavior. In this section, techniques of role playing will be discussed, suggestions for the design of role plays will be made, and a sample format for drink/target behavior refusal training presented.

   Role playing is used for a variety of purposes. The three most important for refusal training are assessment, skill acquisition, and anxiety reduction.

   Step 1. Assessment. People are often unaware of how they behave. It is not uncommon for a client's verbal description of an incident to be entirely different from his or her actual behavior in that situation. Because it is not feasible to observe the client in the actual drink refusal situation, an alternative is to recreate that situation, or at least crucial aspects of it, in the therapist's office. When the client role plays his or her version of what happened, the therapist can learn much about how the client actually operates in a crucial situation and consequently can more accurately assess the nature and extent of the problem. The therapist can observe not only the words the client used in the situation but also the nonverbal components of the interaction, for example, the client's tone of voice, clarity and fluency of speech, facial expression, and bodily stance. Having an accurate picture of the problem is, of course, essential to designing a helpful intervention.

   Step 2. Skill Acquisition. Many clients do not know how to behave appropriately yet assertively in interpersonal situations. Alcoholics, for example, have often had no experience saying "no" when offered a drink. When clients lack the skill to say "no," it is the therapist's job to teach them. When designing the role play, keep in mind that it is an inefficient use of time to try to practice something a person does not know how to do. First the client needs to know what to do, and then the behavior can be practiced or role played. The client can, with the help of the therapist or the partner, decide on the lines to be used in the refusal, or the refusal can be demonstrated or modeled by the therapist. Therapists who work with alcoholics might want to make a videotape of several suitable ways to refuse a drink under a variety of situations.

Step 3. Anxiety Reduction. Sometimes people already have the necessary skills to perform as they would like but are anxious about using them. Practice of the behavior in the less threatening environment of the therapeutic situation can give clients the confidence to perform the behavior in the real world. As always, extra doses of encouragement and reinforcement are called for when the client is anxious.

Role-Playing Techniques

There are a variety of role-playing techniques that can be used in the service of refusal training. In this part of the program, the therapist has an opportunity to be creative in tailoring the combination of techniques to the particular needs of the clients. Some of the most useful role-playing techniques are described below.

Behavioral Rehearsal

The client plays him- or herself and refuses the offer of a drink or an opportunity to engage in the target behavior while the therapist or the partner plays the part of a friend or acquaintance making the offer.

Role Reversal

The client exchanges roles with the therapist or with his or her partner. For example, the therapist might exchange roles with the client, having the client play the part of a friend offering a drink while the therapist plays the client and refuses the drink. By using the role reversal technique two things are accomplished. First, the therapist can demonstrate how to refuse the drink. Second, by watching the client in the role, the therapist can learn how the friend actually behaves and can, thus, do a more accurate job of playing the friend when the roles are switched and it is the therapist's turn to offer the client a drink and the client's turn to refuse.

Coaching

During the rehearsal, the therapist or the partner acts as a coach, instructing or otherwise helping the client with appropriate words to say in the role. For example, the therapist might set up a refusal situation with the partner playing the friend who offers a drink. The therapist then sits close by, so that if the client runs into trouble the therapist can stop the role play and caucus with the client. The two can decide together what the client should say next. Coaching is especially helpful when the client is having great difficulty with the rehearsal, perhaps being distressed by the notion of play acting or unable to think of what to say in the role.

Graded Hierarchy

With the client, a number of refusal situations are created, then arranged in a hierarchy of difficulty, and finally rehearsed starting with the situation that the client views as easiest and proceeding up the hierarchy to the most difficult situation at the top. The more drink refusal is a problem for the client, the more likely working with a hierarchy is to be helpful.

Rehearsing Cognitions

Rather than addressing another person who offers a drink or an opportunity to engage in the targeted behavior, the rehearsal addresses the client's own cognitions. The client's automatic thoughts can be identified by reviewing the Drinking Chains and Target Behavior Charts.

Covert Rehearsal

The client rehearses a refusal situation in his or her head. For example, the client anticipates an upcoming drink refusal situation and rehearses it by imagining him- or herself assertively and confidently refusing the offer. This technique is best used as an adjunct, after the client has rehearsed in vivo in the therapy session.

Videotape

Videotape can be used to great advantage with role playing, for example, to instruct by showing a filmed model displaying the desired refusal behavior, or to show the client how much progress he or she has made by making pre- and posttraining tapes, or to aid in fine-tuning the client's performance.

Suggestions for the Design of Role Plays

Some clients will balk at the notion of role playing, perhaps because they are embarrassed, perhaps because they are afraid they will not do well. It is best to be both encouraging and matter of fact as you introduce the subject; while not ignoring objections, make very little of them. It is reassuring to the client if the therapist appears confident, by saying, for example, "Don't worry, I'll show you how." In order to shape the client's behavior so that you can proceed with the role-play agenda, the first few times a reluctant client does anything that even approximates playing a role, calmly say, "Good job."

Most problems in behavioral rehearsal occur because the therapist did not thoroughly understand the problematic situation. It is very important to be absolutely clear about the refusal situation (who, when, where, how many, etc.) before you set up the role play. Then make the set up as realistic as possible, for example, by having the client stand with one foot on the rung of a chair to simulate a bar, if that is the environmental context to be rehearsed.

It is important, also, that each rehearsal session end on a positive note. To make this happen, a situation may need to be rehearsed many times, and the therapist may need to interrupt the clients to ensure that they do not practice behaviors that are self-defeating or useless. If the therapist informs the clients at the outset that they may be interrupted but "That's okay, we'll just begin again," the clients will very likely take the interruptions in stride.

Finally, whenever possible, include the partner in the rehearsals, because the partner can be of considerable help in the refusal training and because in the active, cognitive-behavioral model therapy is less effective when half of a couple sit and watch while the therapist works with the other half. Clearly, not all partners at all times can be counted on to facilitate learning; giggling, attempting to be funny, and using the rehearsal as an opportunity to make a point or get even are common misdemeanors. Thus, be aware of the partner's mood and alert to possible trouble the partner might cause, and design the role play accordingly.

Silent Technique

The client is asked to role play a drink refusal situation without speaking. This technique might be appropriate in a situation where the client is saying "no" with words, but "yes" with nonverbal behaviors. The silent technique forces a person to focus on nonverbal aspects of behavior.

Mirror Technique

After the client has played a role, another person plays the client's role in order to help the client understand how he or she is seen by others.

Broken Record Technique

One specific technique utilized in drink/target behavior refusal training is called the "broken record" (M. J. Smith, 1975). The broken record is an assertive technique that often comes in handy when someone is trying to sell you something that you do not want, or trying to get you to do something that you do not want to do. Thus, it can be very useful for clients when someone is offering them a drink and they are no longer drinking. The reason for its effectiveness with clients who are refusing alcohol or refusing to engage in a target behavior is twofold. First, for the client refusing alcohol, the technique involves having the client respond to the offer of a drink with a short, concise phrase which is easy to remember and helps him or her stay committed to abstinence by repeating an empowering phrase (e.g., "I am no longer drinking," or "I am a recovering alcoholic"). Second, by using this broken phrase over and over, the person offering the drink usually gets "stumped" quickly and realizes that no matter how forceful he or she is, the refusing party is not going to give in. The same process may be applied to the partner refusing to engage in target behavior. The rules are simple and are presented here briefly. (A more detailed version of the rules, with an example, is found in Forma 8a and 8b.)

Note. For the sake of simplicity, the following steps are stated in terms of refusing a drink only. However, the technique will also apply to most target behaviors and may be used with the partner as well.

Step 1. Have the clients decide on roles; one client is the person refusing and the other is the person offering. The person refusing to drink decides on a short, broken record phrase that represents how he or she feels or thinks about the situation. For example, "I am no longer drinking," or, "I am a recovering alcoholic," or, "I have had problems with alcohol and I don't drink." It is important that the phrase be meaningful to the person refusing the behavior, and that it be short and concise.

Step 2. After deciding on a situation to role play, the offering client begins asking the refusing client if he or she wants a drink. The first time the drink is offered, the refusing client says "no" and gives an honest explanation why the answer is "no." For example, rather than saying, "I am not drinking tonight because I am on medication," the client might say, "I am not drinking because I had a problem with alcohol." Of course, the amount of information to be revealed to the other person will depend on their relationship and the context in which the drink is being offered.

Step 3. The offering client then continues to offer the drink. After the initial refusal and explanation, the refusing client first needs to let the offering client know firmly and politely that he or she understands the offering client's feelings. Next, the refusing client states clearly the broken record phrase—always the EXACT, SAME broken record phrase—repeated as often as necessary. For example, the client would say to the person offering the drink, "Thank you. I know I used to drink with you, but I am no longer drinking," or, "Thanks. I know you'd love it if I drank with you like old times, but I am no longer drinking."

Step 4. The refusing client is to continue to be persistent and unyielding, repeating the broken record phrase as many times as necessary. The client does *not* answer questions as to why he or she is not drinking after the initial explanation because answering the questions or discussing the issue may lead him or her astray.

Step 5. Have the refusing client try to end on a friendly note and possibly suggest an alternative behavior, for example, "I no longer drink, but I would like to get together, how about lunch?"

Step 6. Have clients change roles with each other and repeat the role play. Have both clients practice this skill with a variety of high-risk situations.

Step 7. Vary this technique by having the partner who is offering the drink role play the client's own internal voice that is offering him or her a drink. In this scenario, have the refusing client first share as many of the thoughts as possible that often precede a drinking episode (e.g., "I can have just one," and, "I deserve a drink," and, "I can just drink today and quit again tomorrow") and then have the partner use these phrases to "offer" the client a drink. Have the refusing client utilize the same strategies outlined above to refuse the drink.

General Guidelines for All Role Plays

Below is a list of guidelines for implementing the role plays.

1. Bring to the session a few preset refusal situations to use if you have trouble getting the ball rolling.
2. Have clients write down on a 3 × 5 index card a few high-risk situations that you will later use for role play.
3. Describe the purpose and rationale for role playing and how each client is to participate.

4. Allow the clients to help design the role play so that it becomes as realistic as possible.
5. Include both clients as much as possible. Provide coaching and/or modeling as necessary.
6. Provide positive feedback after each attempt.
7. BE FLEXIBLE!

Exercises

Depending on how receptive the clients are to role playing (most clients take a little while to warm up and feel comfortable), these drink/target behavior refusal skills can be practiced over a couple of sessions. Possible exercises to use after the in-session role plays are as follows.

1. Have clients write down an upcoming high-risk situation that they can role play in the next session.
2. Have clients practice the role play done in session, or another role play with a different technique or situation, at home.
3. Have clients record all situations where they actually refused a drink or refused to engage in the target behavior (regardless of whether refusal was to client's own internal voice or to another person). Have them record their responses to the invitation to drink or engage in the target behavior and bring to the next session to review with the therapist.

TERMINATION OF ACUTE PHASE OF TREATMENT

For therapists using a 20-session model, it is important to discuss with clients the closure of the Acute Phase, what this means with respect to their treatment, and what to expect in the Relapse Prevention Phase. For therapists not adhering to a 20-session model, the following material may be helpful with respect to reviewing progress with clients and planning for a shift in focus from helping clients stop drinking to helping them maintain their abstinence, or relapse prevention.

Rationale

If you are following the 20-session format suggested in this book, the Acute Phase refers to Early and Middle Treatment, Chapters 4 and 6 (as well as work with the communication skills taught in Chapter 5). This phase of treatment and the interventions within are designed to work with clients on achieving abstinence and to help them become aware of the cognitive and behavioral triggers that have led to drinking or engaging in the target behavior in the past. During this phase of treatment, the clients were taught how to identify their automatic thoughts and counter them with thoughts supportive of abstinent behavior. They also examined their coping resources and practiced using new behavioral coping strategies. All of these components were designed to give the clients a solid foundation and a sense of confidence in their ability to remain abstinent. The Relapse Prevention Phase offers the clients a chance to integrate these new concepts and practice the new skills in their daily lives, and introduces further skills to help them maintain abstinence.

If you are not following the 20-session format, take time in therapy to summarize successes and assess further treatment needs. Furthermore, taking time to acknowledge successes may increase compliance and help the clients build confidence in their ability to maintain abstinence.

1. Terminating the Acute Phase has a number of logistical consequences, as well as treatment considerations. The consequences (if you are following the 20-session approach) include the cessation of biweekly meetings and the introduction of a tapered meeting schedule, whereby you meet once a week for 3 weeks, once every other week for 8 weeks, and then after skipping 2 weeks, meet for the last time. Of course, you can adjust this meeting schedule to meet your needs and those of the clients. This schedule was devised in order to offer 20 sessions in 5 months, giving the clients ample time to integrate what they have learned into their daily lives. The tapered approach allows clients the opportunity to try out new skills and still have a chance to come back to therapy to modify or fine-tune these skills. Discussing schedule changes and the impact of these changes on the clients' lives is very important. For example, if you begin meeting less frequently, explore with the clients what they will do with their extra time. This may be a high-risk time for clients, and, if so, it needs to be addressed.

2. Reviewing the treatment thus far and acknowledging successes serves to reinforce the benefits of participating in therapy and working hard on achieving goals. The clients have covered a great deal of territory in a short period of time and it is important to recognize their achievements. The therapist also has an opportunity to review problem areas and decide on the best plan of action for the remainder of therapy.

3. The Relapse Prevention Phase is designed to meet the individual needs of the clients, and while a framework and options for treatment are provided, much of the activity will depend on the clients' needs. Thus, it will be important to take time during this session to prioritize these needs in order to ensure that the clients meet their program goals and maintain their abstinence.

4. We suggest clients have at least 2 weeks of abstinence before

continuing with the program. If they have been unsuccessful in meeting this objective, it is critical to reevaluate their goals, your approach, and any other factors that may be contributing to this behavior (e.g., lack of commitment from the couple). It may be necessary to increase the intensity of the treatment (meet more frequently), assess for underlying depression or other psychiatric conditions that may preclude treatment at this time, evaluate need for medically supervised detoxification, or address marital problems interfering with the alcoholism treatment before proceeding further.

Procedure

In order to terminate the Acute Phase of treatment appropriately and to set the stage for the Relapse Prevention Phase, we suggest the following steps (see the Case Illustration below for an example of how to implement this topic).

Step 1. Summarize the past 12 sessions (if following the 20-session format), or summarize treatment thus far.

Step 2. Have both clients discuss their individual successes and successes in their relationship. Encourage them to give each other feedback and positive reinforcement.

Step 3. Then have both clients determine the areas of focus for the Relapse Prevention Phase. You may need to review the clients' charts with them, looking for patterns and areas of difficulty. If you have been taking notes throughout the program, they may be helpful at this point.

Step 4. Help the clients prioritize their needs for the remainder of the program and write them down. Make note of those issues they would like to continue working on *after* treatment is completed (in the latter part of the Relapse Prevention Phase, clients will be creating a "Recovery Plan" in which they will have the chance to prioritize and plan for dealing with remaining concerns *not* addressed in therapy).

Step 5. Use the Options section of this book (Chapter 8) for ideas or supplementary treatment components. These options are designed to help enhance the clients' sobriety and include rationale, tips, and activities to address the following topics: exercise, smoking cessation, improving sleep, sexuality, nutrition, relaxation, and work. (These are common topics that clients request time to work on, in addition to continuing with interventions introduced in the Acute Phase of treatment.)

Step 6. Explore with clients what the remainder of treatment will look like and share expectations with each other.

Step 7. If following a 20-session model with sessions tapering off, discuss your new meeting schedule and explore any reactions clients have to this change. Ask what they will do with any extra time they have and if they have any concerns about lapsing. Change is often difficult for clients in early stages of recovery. It is important to acknowledge this as a high-risk time and to help clients make plans for preventing a relapse.

Exercises

It may be helpful to give clients at-home exercises that will help them feel connected to the next phase of treatment and support them during this transition, such as the following.

1. Have the clients list the areas they still need to work on, if you were unable to get through all the material in this session, or, if you completed this step, have them prioritize their concerns for the latter half of treatment.

2. Have the clients brainstorm with each other how they might work on their remaining concerns in session and at home.

3. Have the clients share with someone, other than their partner, how the program is going for them so far, what their successes have been, and what they plan on focusing on in the remainder of the program.

Case Illustration: Termination of Acute Phase

In order to bring closure to the Acute Phase of treatment, in which the goal is to help the clients cease drinking and engaging in the target behavior, and to begin the Relapse Prevention Phase, in which the goal is to help the clients maintain their abstinence, the therapist reviews the treatment interventions utilized thus far, and the clients' successes. At this point, Mike has relapsed on one occasion after nearly 3 weeks of abstinence and Beth has relapsed five times. Both clients have been regularly completing their charts, actively employing new communication skills, and practicing alternative cognitive and behavioral coping skills to deal with high-risk situations.

Mike sees his successes as his ability to stay abstinent for 3 weeks prior to his relapse, as well as his willingness to reengage in therapy after the relapse. He acknowledges that he has tried new coping strategies that are helping him, and his relationship with Beth has improved. Beth identifies her successes as learning how to reinforce Mike's abstinent behavior and ceasing to nag him about his past drinking. She also agrees with Mike that their relationship has improved and reports enjoying the pleasant events in which they are engaging. Both Mike and Beth are able to give each other positive feedback regarding their successes.

Mike identifies a couple of areas to improve and focus on during the Relapse Prevention Phase. He reports that his work environment is stressful and that he is often unable to complete all of the work he has been assigned. He also identifies his sexual relationship with Beth to be an ongoing problem area. In general, Mike wants to spend more "time alone" with Beth. Beth reports that she is somewhat "bored" with her nursing job and has been wanting to go back to school for some time. She believes that this step will help her focus more on herself and be less focused on "fixing" Mike. She also agrees with Mike that they need help improving their sexual relationship and, in particular, just learning how to be more intimate with each other. Mike also suggests that Beth needs to look at her "relapses" because she has used caffeine five times since they started the program. Beth is somewhat defensive at first regarding this feedback, but eventually shares that she has not been taking her goal very seriously. She reports that she is willing to "recommit" to abstinence.

The therapist's feedback to Mike regarding areas to focus on include dealing with anger and frustration, as well as developing a stronger, non-drinking, social support network. His thoughts about drinking and his relapse occurred after incidents where he had argued with someone and after he had spent time with drinking friends. The feedback to Beth regarding areas to focus on included recommitting to the goal of abstinence and focusing more on herself and on getting her needs met.

The options from Chapter 8 to be utilized in the Relapse Prevention Phase are sexuality and relaxation. The couple make plans for how they will begin to work on each of these issues both in and out of session. They agree to start by having a conversation before the next session about what is satisfying and unsatisfying about their sexual relationship and then use the next session to identify strategies for working through the difficulties. They also plan another pleasant event. The therapist also presents a tentative plan for how the remainder of treatment will be spent, integrating these treatment goals. The next session will focus on developing a more specific Action Plan for implementing these new goals and interventions.

Before concluding this discussion, the therapist discusses the tapering of the sessions. (Again, the purpose of the tapering is to allow the clients plenty of time, before the termination of therapy, to integrate new skills and bring back to treatment issues with which they are still struggling.) The clients discuss their reactions and make plans for how they will spend their extra time.

RELAPSE PREVENTION
PHASE

CHAPTER 7

Phase IV:
Relapse Prevention

Overview

Evaluation of Progress and Assessment of Abstinence
Building a Support Network
Creating Individualized Action Plans
Implementing Action Plan Interventions

Materials Needed:

♦ Support Network (Form 9)
♦ Action Plans (Form 10)
♦ Exercise Records (Form 3)
♦ Pencils and Clipboards

Recommended number of sessions: 6

Goals: 1. *Evaluate clients' progress and assess abstinence.*
2. *Explore clients' support network and make recommendations for enhancement.*
3. *Prioritize recovery needs at this phase in treatment.*
4. *Create individualized Action Plans for addressing these needs.*

Relapse prevention is a critical phase of any alcoholism treatment program. It provides an opportunity for clients to consolidate gains made during the acute phase of treatment; to continue learning and improving their coping skills, especially in areas where they are still struggling; and to begin preparing for the termination of treatment.

In our approach, we begin by having clients and therapists review the treatment plan and assess the clients' progress thus far. The next step is to

evaluate the clients' existing support networks and make recommendations, as necessary, for improvement. The support network will be extremely important once therapy ends and it is critical that clients have a
stable network in place before termination. The last step is to prioritize
the alcoholic and his or her partner's recovery needs for the remainder of
the program. Once these needs are determined, individualized Action
Plans are developed in order to help clients and therapists focus the
treatment. The following chapter offers treatment options to explore (e.g.,
nutrition and sobriety, sexuality and sobriety, work and sobriety) that may
be helpful when creating the Action Plans.

EVALUATION OF PROGRESS
AND ASSESSMENT OF ABSTINENCE

Before moving on to the relapse prevention interventions, there are two
important topics to address with clients: evaluation of their progress and
assessment of abstinence. The relapse prevention interventions are based
on the assumption that the clients have achieved their goals of abstinence
and intend to maintain abstinence after treatment ends. If this is not the
case, a careful review of the clients' goals, the Behavioral Contract, and
any obstacles to achieving these goals is recommended. We suggest that if
the clients are still having difficulty not drinking or engaging in the target
behavior at this point, they be encouraged to employ all the skills they
have learned thus far and attempt complete abstinence for the 2 weeks
following this discussion. If they are unable to maintain complete abstinence, the overall treatment goals and treatment program should be
evaluated. It may be necessary to increase the length of the Acute Phase,
to discuss with the clients their readiness for behavioral change, or to refer
the clients to a more intensive program.

   One of the unique aspects of this program is the extensive involvement of the alcoholic's partner in treatment. The partner's goals are
afforded as much respect and consideration as the alcoholic's. However,
if at some point, the partner's behavior is impeding the alcoholic's treatment (e.g., the alcoholic is abstinent, but the partner is still engaging in
the target behavior), it will be essential to discuss this with the clients and
decide how to proceed. It may be that the partner needs to adjust his or
her goals, recommit to the stated goals, and/or examine and modify
sabotaging behaviors. These points also hold true for the partner who is
also alcoholic and has chosen alcohol as his or her target behavior.
However, if the partner continues to abuse alcohol, he or she will need to
be referred to a more intensive treatment.

Moderate Drinking?

At some point during the program, whether during the Acute Phase, Relapse Prevention Phase, or Termination Phase, the alcoholic may bring up the issue of moderate drinking. In essence, the client states that instead of not drinking at all, he or she would prefer to drink occasionally. This announcement may very likely be followed by a convincing argument, whereby the client attempts to establish his or her ability to "handle it."

If the client brings up the idea during treatment, the response depends on your treatment philosophy. In the approach suggested in this book, the response is simple; that is, if the client wishes to continue in the program, he or she must agree to complete abstinence. The reasons for this response are twofold. First, the vast majority of research on alcoholism maintains that abstinence, although quite difficult to maintain at times, is the optimum goal for people with severe drinking problems. Second, the agreement the client made upon entering treatment was to remain abstinent throughout the program and it is important to uphold this agreement. It is certainly valuable and critical, however, to explore why the client wishes to change this agreement at this time. Additionally, we recommend including the partner in this discussion and making sure he or she has time to express reactions to the alcoholic's announcement. Often, a little "reality check" from the partner ends up playing a major role in the alcoholic's decision.

If your clientele includes problem drinkers who have not reached the addictive state of the disorder, and you believe they can successfully learn to moderate their drinking behavior, we suggest you address the clients' wishes appropriately. Most of the treatment components in this manual are applicable to maintenance of moderate drinking, with a little creativity and flexibility on the part of the therapist. However, it will be critical for the therapist to evaluate the clients' ability to moderate their drinking continually and suggest abstinence if there is any doubt.

Lapse or Relapse

Another important discussion with clients, once they have achieved abstinence, is how a lapse or relapse will be handled. A "lapse" is a term coined by Marlatt and Gordon (1985) to refer to the singular occurrence or act of drinking (or any behavior in question) following a period of abstinence, whereas a "relapse" is the "full return to the former behavior" (p. 32). The purpose of distinguishing between a lapse and a relapse is because clients often set themselves up for a long and difficult journey back to treatment once they start drinking again. This occurs because of a set of cognitions that leads the client to believe that once they violate the rule of abstinence (i.e., have a drink), they are doomed. For many alcoholics, the term "relapse" has a connotation that a person has returned to alcoholic drinking, has "blown it," and is doomed to continue drinking. With this thinking, the alcoholic will often decide that because he or she already "blew it," he or she might as well "keep drinking." Marlatt and Gordon introduced the term "lapse" (which can also be thought of as a "slip") to help these types of thinkers realize that if they have *one* drink, or *one* drinking episode, it doesn't mean that they "blew it"; thus they don't have to return to heavy, regular drinking. Rather, they can view this lapse as a mistake or an ineffective coping response, and can get back on track and become abstinent again *immediately.*

An important note about making a distinction between a lapse and a relapse with clients is that most alcoholics initially interpret the distinction of a lapse as permission to drink every so often. Furthermore, significant others initially respond to the distinction with fear that the alcoholics will hear it as license to drink occasionally (they have usually caught on to the alcoholic thinking by now!). Thus, if using this concept, it is important to explore clients' initial reactions, as well as checking in with them later in treatment because sometimes this thinking starts to kick in later on. It can be a very useful and empowering concept for the alcoholic who is used to shaming him- or herself when they make mistakes or succumb to a high-risk situation.

Regardless of whether you introduce the concept of a "lapse," it is important to discuss your plan to handle a drinking episode should it occur, as well as a return to the target behavior by the partner. The couple should come to some agreement *together* as to how they will deal with drinking or engagement in the target behavior. This is one issue where having the partner abstaining from a target behavior is particularly helpful. Significant others are often very fearful and controlling when the topic of relapse arises. When having to face the possibility of their own relapse, a greater degree of empathy and understanding often emerges. In general, our recommendation is to use the lapse or relapse as a learning opportunity, analyze it with the Drinking Chain II (or Target Behavior Chart II), and explore alternative coping strategies. If a patient continues to drink or continues to have relapses, once again, we recommend reviewing the treatment goals, the Behavioral Contract, and the possibility of referral to a higher level of care (e.g., day treatment or residential treatment).

Discussion of Progress

Discussing progress with clients can be done intermittently throughout treatment and is particularly helpful as the therapist moves from one phase of treatment to another (e.g., Middle Treatment Phase to the Relapse Prevention Phase). It is particularly helpful at this transition (moving into the Relapse Prevention Phase) so that clients can refocus on treatment goals and recommit to treatment. Being in treatment for alcoholism is difficult for both the alcoholic and the partner. It requires a great deal of in-session and out-of-session work and can become draining. It is important for clients to receive feedback on their progress and successes, as well as be able to give feedback regarding what is working for them in treatment and what is not. An example of how a discussion of progress can be beneficial is in the case of the clients who are maintaining abstinence but are having a difficult time identifying triggers on their self-monitoring charts. In this case, the therapist may first acknowledge the abstinence despite the difficulties identifying triggers. Then, the therapist and clients can decide to spend more time on this skill, present the information in a different manner, or simply focus on helping the clients learn general coping skills that can be beneficial regardless of the triggers.

Further rationale for discussing the importance of feedback is addressed by Urban and Ford (1971), who believe that psychotherapy is a "problem-solving approach." They point out that incorporating a "feedback loop" into the psychotherapy process is advantageous in identifying and making modifications when it becomes clear that "the objectives that have been sought are not being fulfilled" (p. 8). Thus, taking time during a session to discuss clients' progress not only increases the chance of early identification of unfulfilled objectives, but also teaches the clients the value of stopping along the way and evaluating their own decisions and actions, in order to optimize their chances of success.

BUILDING A SUPPORT SYSTEM

Although this topic could easily have been included in the previous section on coping resources, we have presented it here to highlight its importance in recovery from alcoholism. The purpose of this section is to focus specifically on the skill of building a strong support network.

Rationale

One factor that has been studied extensively in the mental health field is "social support" and its effect on treatment outcome (Oyabu & Garland, 1987). The findings have been relatively consistent overall; that is, when one has the perception of a strong social support network, there is a greater likelihood of successful treatment outcome and maintenance of change.

These findings have held true in the substance abuse field as well (Gordon & Zrull, 1991; Oyabu & Garland, 1987). It is interesting to note that, in general, the research indicates that it is the "perception" of a strong support system, rather than the actual existence or availability of support, that influences outcome. Although this may be the case, we suggest that you explore not only the clients' *perception* of social support, but the actual *availability of this support,* and the clients' *willingness to receive the support.*

1. Social support may mean something different to each person. Therefore, it is important to take time with clients to determine what social support means to them. One definition that we found particularly helpful is by Caplan (1974), who suggested that when people have social support, they are mobilized to action and provided with necessary resources to do so. Encouraging a friend to get into action and get to an AA meeting or to pick up the phone when craving a drink is an important part of social support. In addition, providing either material resources (e.g., transportation, money) or providing encouragement to a friend to tap into his or her own psychological resources (e.g., courage, strength, hope) are also valuable aspects of social support.

Lastly, a social support system that provides affection and affirmation to the client is critical. The road of recovery is often difficult and involves hard work. Hugs and "pats of the back" along the way are encouraging and meaningful. In addition, having friends and family provide positive affirmation and acknowledgment of success is very important. As suggested in the Procedure section below, each of these components of social support should be reviewed with clients to determine the adequacy of their support networks.

2. For many alcoholics, years of drinking have led to a "support group" comprised of other alcoholics. Often these drinking buddies are only fair-weather friends; that is, when the alcohol is gone, so is the friendship. Becoming abstinent represents a significant loss for most alcoholics in treatment, who are not only giving up what has come to be their best friend and ready companion, alcohol, but also losing their circle of friends and acquaintances who shared a compelling interest in alcohol. These feelings of loss are important to explore because they can often trigger drinking urges.

3. It is important to explain to clients that making a public commitment to change and enlisting social support enhances the chances of success. Thus, we encourage clients to let their friends and family know about their abstinence and to ask for support when appropriate.

Procedure

Step 1. Begin by discussing what "support" actually means to the clients. Inquire as to what they find helpful when upset, depressed, or anxious, or when tempted to drink or engage in the target behavior.

Step 2. Have both clients, individually, generate a list of people or groups (e.g., church, AA) they can call on when they need support, using Form 9. The couple can also generate a separate list of people or groups they consider supportive of them as a couple, if different from their lists as individuals. When the clients have named everyone that they can think of, go back over the lists to make sure that they do not include any drinking companions who will not, in fact, provide support if alcohol is not present (if applicable, apply this to target behavior). Have the couple challenge each other as to the reality of their responses to this latter point. For example, if the alcoholic client says that his friend John will be there for him "no matter what," check in with his partner to see whether she agrees that John is not just a "drinking buddy," or if she believes that it would be difficult for her husband to spend time with John because of his drinking. The purpose of including the partner is to get another perspective on the supportive nature of the friendship, as well as to help the couple learn to be supportive of one another, even when challenging one another.

Step 3. Considering the definition of social support mentioned in the Rationale, important aspects of the clients' support systems to review include (1) whether the support has an affective component, (2) whether the support is positively affirming, (3) whether the support serves to mobilize the individual when necessary, (4) whether the support empowers the individual to call on internal resources, and (5) whether the support provides material resources when necessary or appropriate. Thus, when reviewing the clients' lists of supportive people or groups, inquire about the *quality* of this support. The therapist can explore the affective component of the existing social support by asking how emotionally satisfying their support network is and can explore the affirmative nature of the support by asking about the degree of positive affirmation the clients receive from their family and friends. Additionally, it is important to explore whether this support encourages the clients to utilize their own personal resources or encourages dependency on others. Lastly, inquiry into the availability of aid (material or financial) when clients are in need is important, especially for this population, who often use up these resources while drinking. This exploration will give you and the clients an extensive picture of the strengths and weaknesses of their support network, which you may then work with throughout the program.

Step 4. It may become clear that despite the available support, clients have a difficult time asking for the support they need. Thus, ascertain how well the clients can actually ask for the support needed. The therapist might already have a good guess, given the clients' behavior in previous sessions. If not, ask the clients to tell how they ask for support. In addition, set up a role play of a situation in which the clients ask the therapist and/or each other for support.

Step 5. If it appears that the clients need to learn this skill, the following exercise provides a means for the clients to learn and to practice asking for help.

1. First, go over the following guidelines for asking for support:
   a. Set up an appropriate time to ask for the support (e.g., have client ask his or her friend first if this is a good time to talk, or schedule an appointment with the friend). This will help ensure that the client has the other person's attention.
   b. Have client be specific about telling the friend (or whomever) what it is that he or she wants. For example, "I just want you to listen," or, "I could use your help in figuring out some options," or, "I need a hug."
2. With the clients, generate some examples of times when they would like support. Then role play those situations.
3. Fill in the remaining columns of Form 9, listing beside each name how and when they can expect support from this person, and, in the last column, the person's telephone number.

Case Illustration: Support Network

The therapist begins exploring the issue of having a support network by asking the couple what "support" means to each of them. Mike describes support as "having someone to do things with, other than drinking," as well as "financial help." Beth describes support as primarily "having someone to talk to when she is upset." Having heard Beth's description, Mike acknowledges that having someone to talk with is sometimes helpful or supportive as well. The couple then generates a list of people and groups they feel are supportive of them and, in particular, supportive of Mike's abstinence. Mike's list includes Beth, the therapist, his sister, and his friend Paul. Beth's list includes two friends, her sister, church, her two sons, and her parents. The therapist notes that Beth did not include Mike on her list and she responds that she "didn't even think of him." She reports feeling embarrassed that she did not include him and promptly writes his name down. The therapist helps Beth to see that it takes time to start viewing the relationship in a different light. Her willingness to include Mike as a source of support is an important step.

The therapist then asks each partner to review the other's list and give feedback to one another regarding the supportiveness of the person/group listed. Beth immediately challenges Mike regarding his friend Paul. She states that although Paul might say he's supportive, he always drinks around Mike. Mike is defensive in response and states that Paul "might be an alcoholic himself," but he is also a good friend. Mike challenges Beth on having her sister on the list because he feels that her sister was not supportive of their marriage in the first place and is certainly not very positive about their couple therapy.

These challenges lead the therapist to explore with the couple the quality of the support networks they each have and what aspects of these relationships they find supportive. When reviewing the quality of the support, Mike realizes that with Beth and his sister, he feels that he receives affection, caring, concern, and positive affirmation. From the therapist, Mike feels he receives caring and positive affirmation. Other than the therapist, none of the relationships provide Mike with support for using his own internal resources to help himself, nor are they relationships where he feels he can count on the other to provide material resources (in particular, money) when he needs them. He also realizes that although Paul is "fun" to be with, there is not much else that the relationship offers him and that most of the fun was when they were drinking together. Beth's relationships appear to be more fulfilling, providing her with affection, positive affirmation, empowerment, and material resources. She does note, however, that she has withdrawn from most of these people, as well as church, over the past year as Mike's drinking has escalated and she has become more controlling of his behavior and the activities in which they participated. Mike also acknowledges that he has lost touch with a few friends over the years and does not really have any "buddies" with whom he could spend time and not drink.

Both partners explore how they could go about making changes to enhance their support networks. Beth agrees to call one of her friends and have lunch with her. Additionally, she decides to call her sister and share the positive aspects of the therapy with her, rather than just complaining about Mike, which she is accustomed to doing. Mike agrees to try an AA meeting, as well as return to the local gym. He intends to meet some new people with whom he could be friends.

The therapist then explores with the couple how they could be more supportive of each other. Mike states that Beth could make time to spend with him alone on the weekends, rather than always with the boys. Beth states that Mike could pay more attention to her when she is talking about her job. (Note: When issues regarding communication surface, introducing skills from the Communication Skills chapter may be appropriate.) Before the session ends, the therapist has the clients agree to very specific actions they will take over the next week with respect to the behavioral changes they have agreed on (e.g., going to the gym twice, having lunch with one friend, going to one AA meeting).

12-Step Programs as Support Systems

Traditionally in alcoholism treatment, participation in 12-step programs (AA and Al-Anon) is recommended as an adjunct to psychotherapy and for long-term support. Therefore, discussing whether the clients' support system includes (now or in the future) a 12-step program is important. It is helpful to take time to discuss how this cognitive-behavioral treatment approach is compatible with the 12-step programs, because, initially, it may not appear to be. The approach that we have found useful is first to address one of the main philosophies of AA; that is, alcoholics are powerless over alcohol and that their lives have become unmanageable as a consequence of drinking. In order to help the clients bridge the gap between the philosophy of the program presented in this book and that of AA, point out that in the 12-step program, the alcoholic is powerless over alcohol, but *not* powerless over sobriety or his or her behaviors. The present program focuses on the latter point in that it teaches clients how to identify the behaviors that may lead to drinking and replace them with behaviors that support abstinence. Additionally, you may want to remind the clients of an AA slogan, "identify, don't compare," to reinforce the concept that they may use the components of both approaches that are helpful to them.

Al-Anon espouses that the coalcoholic (the partner) did not cause the alcoholism, cannot control it, and cannot cure it, and encourages participants to explore their "enabling" behaviors. Although the present program does not use the term "enabling," it is concerned with the partner's behaviors that are "in reaction" to the alcoholic. Although the partner's intention may be to provide support, reactive responses are often destructive to the individuals and the relationship. Thus, we challenge the partner to identify which of his or her behaviors are reinforcing the alcoholic's drinking and which are reinforcing abstinence. It may be important to emphasize that although a behavior reinforces drinking, it does not mean that it causes drinking. Overall, we are attempting to teach clients that the way that they react to one another may trigger (not cause) urges or thoughts to drink and that learning new behaviors may trigger thoughts that are incompatible with drinking and thus supportive of abstinence. Furthermore, the inclusion of a target behavior allows the partners to learn how to focus on themselves again, rather than expending most of their energy on the alcoholic. This approach is consistent with Al-Anon's position that encourages the co-alcoholic to learn to cope more effectively.

Exercises

1. Most of the interventions in this section, Building a Support System, may be easily extended to at-home exercises for the couple. For example, have clients write down more extensive lists of their individual support networks and how those can be counted on for help, as well as lists of their supports as a couple.

2. As another possible assignment, have the couple examine in depth the quality of their support networks, either during a conversation with each other or in written form.

3. These exercises must be individualized for the clients, depending on their needs, but, if relevant, have both clients practice asking for help from their friends or family, including from each other, especially if this is a difficult task for them.

4. If relevant, give clients an assignment to attend an AA and/or Al-Anon meeting before the next session.

5. If relevant, give clients an assignment to participate in an activity that will enhance their support network, for example, an activity that they have "been meaning to do for a long time," such as attend church or temple, spend time with family, or make a new friend.

The therapist and clients, together, can be creative in exploring activities and assignments that may be helpful to the couple in extending and enhancing their support networks.

CREATING INDIVIDUALIZED ACTION PLANS

As mentioned in the previous chapter, it is important to review the clients' progress and explore remaining concerns for treatment. This will help the therapist and clients develop a focus for the Relapse Prevention Phase. In the section in Chapter 6, Termination of Acute Phase of Treatment, we recommended having clients write down their lists of concerns, or areas they wished to work on, in the time remaining in treatment. After reviewing the clients' prioritized list of concerns, decide which concerns you will address during the remainder of treatment and which concerns you will include in the clients' Recovery Plans to work on after the completion of therapy. Then, we recommend using the Action Plan (Form 10) to organize your treatment goals for the Relapse Prevention Phase.

Rationale

The purpose of the Action Plan is twofold. One objective is to prioritize the clients' needs for the remainder of the program and organize your time to ensure that these needs are adequately met. The second objective is to teach the clients the process of setting goals, deciding on strategies for achieving those goals, and setting target dates for completion of the goals.

1. Because the clients often have a number of concerns and problems that they want to address during treatment, it can be helpful to organize these objectives using a form such as the Action Plan. Discussing the clients' concerns and prioritizing them can also help the clients become more realistic about setting goals and can uncover the time it takes to address each problem area adequately. It is not uncommon to find clients who want to quit drinking, quit smoking, lose weight, change their diet, and begin an exercise program—all at the same time. Using a goal-setting strategy such as the Action Plan will be advantageous with such clients to help prevent relapse and to help teach them the benefits of taking one problem at time and building on each success until the ultimate goal is obtained. By approaching one's problems in this matter, self-efficacy can be strengthened (Bandura, 1977a) and the likelihood of taking on another challenge increased.

2. Marlatt and Gordon (1985) point out the benefits of making proximal goals, or subgoals, rather than setting one large goal. One such benefit is that when a setback occurs, it can be viewed as a "subgoal problem," rather than a "total breakdown" (p. 226). This view is an important one for alcoholics who often see problems as black or white and engage in all-or-nothing thinking. That is, if the alcoholic has a drink after a period of abstinence, he or she is likely to say, "What the heck, I already blew it, I might as well get drunk." Note that this perspective is consistent with Marlatt and Gordon's (1985) distinction between lapse and relapse described earlier in this chapter. By looking at a single drinking episode as a lapse rather than a relapse, or viewing a setback in other behavioral goals as merely a subgoal problem instead of complete failure, clients are able to acknowledge that mistakes do not necessarily mean that all their efforts are of no value and that it is time to give up. Instead, the clients learn how to deal with mistakes and quickly get back on track in meeting their desired objectives.

3. Teaching clients the process of goal setting, which includes decid-ing on strategies and setting target dates to achieve these goals, can be one

of the most valuable components of treatment. This is especially significant for alcoholics, many of whom have difficulty delaying gratification.
As McCrady, Dean, Dubreuil, and Swanson (1985) point out when
describing the "Problem Drinkers' Project," goal setting enables the clients
to learn to (1) plan ahead, (2) contemplate various methods for achieving
short-term goals, and (3) recognize that these short-term objectives lead
to long-term achievements. Clients often report that practicing goal-setting skills and learning how to cope with their impatience are practical,
useful tools they can apply in many areas of their lives.

Procedure

The Action Plan (Form 10) is a tool that helps clients organize their goals
for the Relapse Prevention Phase of treatment, set priorities for these goals,
and decide on strategies for accomplishing them. The following guidelines
are offered to assist in completing the Action Plan (remember to engage
the couple in working together as much as possible to generate ideas, as
well as to give positive reinforcement to each other).

Step 1. Begin by reviewing with the clients how the charts, communication skills, pleasant events, coping skills, support network enhancement, and any additional treatment components have been helpful to them
in maintaining their abstinence and in reaching their treatment goals.

Step 2. Take the clients' lists of concerns from the previous session
and help them decide which ones to work on during the next four or five
sessions. (Be realistic about how much you can accomplish in the time
allotted). Additionally, *we recommend that the focus of these concerns be
limited to those problems that are currently jeopardizing their sobriety, or
may put them at risk for relapse in the future* (e.g., stress at work,
difficulties with sleep, poor nutrition).

Step 3. Help the clients prioritize these problem areas and make note
of the concerns that you will not have time to address (these will be
included in the Recovery Plan to be addressed after the program has
ended).

Step 4. Starting with the first priority, help the clients restate their
concern into a goal. For example, if the concern is "I still have difficulty
relaxing when I get home from work," the goal might be "learn relaxation
techniques that I can use when I get home from work." (Note: You may
choose to work with one client at a time to complete his or her Action
Plan or alternate working with one client on his or her first goal, then
working on the other client's first goal, etc.)

Step 5. Next, have the couple brainstorm strategies for achieving their goals. These strategies may include plans for activities in therapy sessions as well as out of session (e.g., at home, at work). After generating a few ideas, and giving your feedback, decide on a list of activities clients are willing to do. (See the sample Action Plan in Figure 7.1.)

Step 6. Once the strategies are determined, decide which sessions will be used to work on the goal at hand and what the target date and outcome will be. To address a concern adequately, you may need only one session (e.g., teaching relaxation skills) or three sessions (e.g., teaching smoking cessation strategies). The target date may be during the program or after the program has ended, depending on the goal. The outcome is a statement about what the clients hope to achieve by the target date; for example, "I will be a nonsmoker on January 13th," or "I will be healthier and I will be happy that I finally quit," or "I will be using relaxation techniques three times a week after work by January 20th."

Step 7. *Most importantly, the goals, strategies, and outcome must be specific and measurable.* For example, it is *not* recommended to have a goal like "getting along better with my wife" because it is neither specific

---

PRIORITY: 1

PROBLEM AREA: Stress after work

GOAL: To learn how to relax when I get home from work

STRATEGIES: In session: 1. Learn relaxation
                                    techniques

              Out of session: 1. Practice techniques

                                  2. Buy a relaxation tape

                                  3. Ask my husband and
                                     children to give me 20
                                     minutes to be alone
                                     when I get home

WORK ON DURING SESSIONS: 14 and 15

TARGET DATE AND OUTCOME: I will use relaxation techniques three times a week when I get off work by January 13th; I will buy a relaxation tape by January 7th; I will start asking for "alone time" each day that I need it by January 13th.

FIGURE 7.1. Sample Action Plan.

nor measurable. A better goal would be "go out on a date once a week with my wife and have conversations with her at dinner."

Step 8. Decide with clients if it will be helpful to continue the Drinking Chain II and Target Behavior Chart II, as well as to continue with the pleasant events. Clients may choose to continue using these tools, but not review them regularly in therapy sessions.

Exercises

1. If you were unable to complete the Action Plans in session, you may opt to have clients complete them or add to them at home.

2. Remind clients, if they are completing their Action Plans at home, to work together to get support and feedback from one another.

IMPLEMENTING ACTION PLAN INTERVENTIONS

We recommend that about five sessions be spent on interventions specific to reaching the goals included in the Action Plans. The structure is flexible and the following recommendations, based on our experience during this phase of treatment, are offered as guidelines.

Guidelines

1. Continue to be realistic about how much can be covered in one session. It is very important to follow through with each intervention agreed on and with each goal included in the Action Plan. Thus, if time is limited, it is better to address the scarcity of time and modify the Action Plan than try to cram everything into the five sessions or to disregard any of the stated goals.

2. Have the couple negotiate the amount of time to be spent on each individual and be mindful of this agreement. As the therapist, you may need to facilitate this negotiation, especially if one client is more needy than the other or if one partner feels less deserving of time because the stated focus of treatment is the alcoholism. These issues need to be considered and the importance of the partner's participation reiterated when necessary.

3. Integrate skills covered in the Acute Phase of treatment throughout this Relapse Prevention Phase. For example, continue to provide feedback to the couple on their communication skills, continue to explore high-risk situations and triggers, and inquire about their use of cognitive and behavioral coping strategies.

4. Decide on at-home exercises collectively and again, make sure to follow up on any tasks assigned.

5. Don't be surprised if clients have a lapse, miss sessions, or forget homework. The clients have been in the maintenance phase of treatment, highlighted by consolidating gains, stabilizing behavior change, and preventing relapse. Clients with addictive behaviors often spiral back through earlier stages during their recovery (Prochaska, DiClemente, & Norcross, 1992). It is possible that changes in the schedule and the focus of treatment may be experienced as distressing, which in turn may lead to temporary backsliding. Drinking (or resuming target behavior) during this phase may indicate a client's desire to test his or her control once again; it may be a reaction to a lessening of intensity of treatment (if you are meeting less often), or it may indicate that the clients are taking on too much at one time. There may be numerous other triggers for drinking during this phase and such incidents need to be assessed carefully. One strategy for examining a drinking episode is to use the Drinking Chain II, which helps analyze the episode from a number of perspectives—that is, explore with the client who he or she was with; what he or she was doing, thinking, and feeling; and what were the consequences of the drinking. Once again, use the partner to give feedback and explore his or her thoughts and feelings about the drinking episode. This guideline also applies to the partner who has engaged in his or her target behavior after a period of abstinence.

6. Encourage clients to continue to enhance their coping resources and build their support networks, whether this means participation in self-help groups, meeting new friends, taking risks to be more intimate with each other, or reaching out to existing friends and family.

7. Earlier in this chapter, we recommended that the goals pursued in the Action Plan be ones that will enhance sobriety. If you follow this recommendation, it is important to review with clients how their pursuit, or successful completion, of a goal, has enhanced their sobriety. For example, if a client's goal is to eat more nutritious foods (e.g., more fruits and vegetables, less fat), then it is important continually to explore how changes in diet affect abstinence behavior. If the client's goal is to improve his or her sexual relationship (e.g., have sex more often and communicate likes and dislikes more often), it would be important to inquire about the impact of any accomplishments in this area on sobriety, as well as how sobriety affects this area.

Exercises

At-home exercises will be individually designed at this phase in treatment.

CHAPTER 8

Treatment Options for Implementation during the Relapse Prevention Phase

OVERVIEW

Nutrition and Sobriety
Sexuality and Sobriety
Sleep and Sobriety
Work and Sobriety
Exercise and Sobriety
Smoking Cessation and Sobriety
Relaxation and Sobriety

Materials Needed:
  ♦ Pencils and Clipboards

Recommended number of sessions: to be integrated into the Relapse Prevention Phase of treatment (see Chapter 7)

Goals: 1. Provide clients with options for treatment interventions during the Relapse Prevention Phase.

2. Teach clients effective coping skills in the areas of nutrition, sexuality, sleep, work, exercise, smoking cessation and/or relaxation, which will serve to enhance the quality of their lives and sobriety.

This chapter briefly covers seven topics that the therapist and clients may choose to focus on in the Relapse Prevention Phase of treatment. The topics (nutrition, sexuality, sleep, work, exercise, smoking cessation, and relaxation) address areas of the clients' lives that are often affected by drinking. In the Relapse Prevention Phase of treatment outlined in this book, clients are to choose behaviors, or areas of their lives (e.g., work) that need improvement, with the notion that improvement of these behaviors or areas of their lives will help them maintain abstinence. The topics are each covered briefly, but contain background information that may be helpful, especially with respect to the relationship between the topic and alcoholism. In addition, suggested in-session and out-of-session exercises are included.

Note. Portions of the following text have been adapted from Ann Geller's (1991a) book, *Restore Your Life: A Living Plan for Sober People,* with permission from the author.

NUTRITION AND SOBRIETY

Eating well has many benefits for a healthy lifestyle and for enhancing sobriety. Eating a well-balanced diet can decrease cravings for alcohol, improve energy levels, promote a steady mood, increase levels of concentration, and increase enjoyment and relaxation (Geller, 1991a). The good news for an alcoholic who changes his or her diet is that benefits can be felt relatively quickly. Changing one's diet is also more rewarding if both partners commit to making the change. For couples who have not had a meal together for quite awhile, cooking and eating healthy foods together can restore and strengthen their relationship.

Once both partners see what they are eating, they can begin to make changes to their diets. Start with changing one meal at a time. For instance, have the couple plan a healthy dinner together. Magazines such as *Vegetarian Times* and *Cooking Light* are helpful resources for recipes and other cooking ideas.

As the clients begin to alter their diets, it will be important that they have knowledge about good eating habits. Three central principles of good eating are (1) vary the types of food consumed, (2) adhere to regular mealtimes and planned snacks, and (3) eat in moderation (Geller, 1991a, pp. 272–273).

For the alcoholic client, there are additional factors to consider regarding nutritional health. First of all, as a result of chronic, heavy drinking, the alcoholic's nutritional status is most likely poor. Alcohol causes cell membranes throughout the body to become "leaky"; thus, many important nutrients are not absorbed. Instead, these nutrients are leaked into the extracellular fluid and eliminated. Consequently, even if the alcoholic has been eating well, he or she may not have been absorbing the proteins and minerals essential for good health.

It may be helpful to refer your client to a physician, who can properly evaluate the client's nutritional status, determine any problems with changing his or her diet, and/or suggest any food supplements or vitamins that may be beneficial. (We recommend that the physician be knowledgeable about alcoholism and the effects of this disorder.)

Of course, as with any lifestyle change, it is important to begin the change process slowly and build from a foundation that is comfortable. Quick changes to new behavior generally do not last and, if they fail, may even be a trigger that prompts drinking behavior.

Exercises

1. One of the first steps in addressing this topic is to discuss with clients their current eating patterns and how changes in these patterns may enhance their sobriety.

2. Clients may find it helpful to keep a "food diary" for a couple of weeks to get a more accurate account of what they are eating (type of food) and how much they are eating (quantity and amount of nutrients, fats, carbohydrates, etc.). From the diary, the clients can decide what changes they would like to make and how they will go about making the changes.

3. Depending on the expertise of the therapist, he or she may provide feedback to the clients regarding their eating patterns or refer the clients to a nutritionist.

4. Clients may also decide to cut back or abstain from particular foods (e.g., high-fat foods, sweets) and use the cognitive-behavioral strategies from the previous chapters to make changes.

5. Have clients take note (written or verbal) of emotional and physical changes that appear as they change their nutritional habits. For example, inquire whether clients notice increased or decreased energy, improved sleep, or improved concentration.

SEXUALITY AND SOBRIETY

This section reviews important information regarding the connection between alcohol abuse and sexual problems. Some suggestions are offered as a means for couples to begin to deal with these problems. Based on the severity of the client's problems and the expertise of the therapist, a determination can be made as to whether the clients need to be referred out for further treatment.

Alcohol Use and Sexual Functioning for Men

About 50% of alcoholic males seeking treatment report problems with sexual potency (Geller, 1991a). These problems stem from a variety of causes. Alcohol use interferes with the ability to produce testosterone, which can lead, in turn, to decreased interest in sex, as well as difficulties with sexual performance. It also causes increased levels of estradiol, which can contribute to erectile dysfunction (Tiefer & Melman, 1989). Alcohol effects the nerves in the penis that carry sensation to the brain, which may lead to difficulties in achieving or maintaining an erection (Geller, 1991a). These physiological changes begin to reverse when alcohol is no longer being ingested. This reversal can take from 2 weeks to a full year depending on the amount of damage that the body has sustained. If after 3 to 6 months of abstinence your client cannot achieve a full erection or masturbate to orgasm, it is wise to refer him to a physician.

Transitory erectile dysfunction may occur for some men at the beginning of sobriety if they have never before experienced sex when not intoxicated (McCarthy, 1992). These men will need to learn sexual arousal patterns that are based on sensations and stimulation rather than on alcohol consumption. It is particularly helpful to let them know that this dysfunction is temporary and is a natural part of the transition to sobriety.

Alcohol Use and Sexual Functioning for Women

Women coming into treatment for alcoholism also suffer problems with the ability to become aroused and to achieve orgasm. Alcohol harms the nerve endings around the clitoris, causing reduced sensation. Arousal and lubrication are diminished, as is sensory feedback that leads to orgasm (Geller, 1991a). There is a paradoxical response, however, to the alcohol: While women's physiological functioning may be impaired, their self-reported subjective arousal levels are increased. Thus, drinking women may desire a sexual encounter, but ultimately find it unsatisfying. Furthermore, as with men, it may take women 6 months to a year to get used to having sober sex.

Exercises

The following exercises are suggested for helping clients use the interpersonal skills learned in treatment to enhance their sexual relationship.

1. Encourage the clients to use the communication skills they learned in this program to talk frankly about sex (e.g., assertive expression of wants and desires, and active listening). Communicating directly and giving positive reinforcement to each other may lead to greater intimacy and a more fulfilling sexual experience.

2. Have the clients explore new problem-solving techniques to find solutions that allow each partner's needs to be meet.

3. Encourage the clients to participate in pleasurable, nonsexual physical contact and to continue to spend time doing pleasant events

together. Again, these activities may increase the couple's sense of intimacy and increase their desire to be sexual with one another.

4. If clients are reporting sexual difficulties, a thorough assessment indicated. The difficulties may be transitory as a result of the alcohol use, and/or may need special therapeutic attention. If the therapist is competent in assessment of sexual functioning and in providing therapy for such difficulties, he or she may proceed with this intervention; otherwise, a referral may be necessary.

SLEEP AND SOBRIETY

Alcoholics may find that they experience sleep disturbances in early recovery. Sleep disturbances are very common in people who stop drinking and may last a few weeks to a few months.

Alcohol intake interrupts the natural sleep pattern. Instead of falling asleep in a progressive, natural way, a person who drinks to excess will often "pass out." The normal stages of restful sleep, including the important rapid-eye-movement (REM) sleep, are bypassed, and, as a consequence, the drinker will generally not feel revitalized after sleep but, rather, tired and unrested.

Some of the side effects a client may experience as a result of quitting drinking, especially in the early stages, include difficulty falling and staying asleep, difficulty staying awake throughout the day, and nightmares or disturbed sleep.

It is important for the alcoholic to allow his or her body to get accustomed to being substance free. This means allowing the body to reestablish normal sleep rhythms. In general, sleep medications are not recommended for alcoholics in early sobriety because these medications change sleep patterns and disrupt dreaming. In addition, sleep medications may have a rebound effect: the alcoholic will have a more difficult time falling and staying asleep the following night. This disrupted cycle may lead to abuse of sleeping medications or may, in fact, trigger a lapse back into the familiar sedation of drinking. If a client is presenting with these symptoms and they do not resolve as a result of continued abstinence, he or she may need to be referred to a physician. In addition, if a client's sleep problems are interfering with their functioning and pose a threat to sobriety, a referral may be in order.

The eight hints Geller (1991a, pp. 262–264) recommends to help the alcoholic in early recovery include the following:

1. *Go to bed and get up at regular times.* Help the alcoholic and his or her partner to establish a workable and consistent bedtime and waking time in order to reinitiate regular biological rhythms.

2. *Avoid activities or substances that may delay sleep.* In order to maximize a natural flow into sleep, most of us should avoid stimulants within 4 hours of established bedtime. Included in this category are nicotine, caffeine (coffee, tea, colas, and chocolate), and any illegal stimulant drugs.

3. *Take a warm bath or shower before bed.* The combined effects of heat and water of a warm bath or shower can induce sleep rhythms in the brain and produce a naturally relaxed and drowsy feeling.

4. *Exercise regularly.* Regular exercise is a wonderful way to promote good health and natural sleep. Make sure there are 4 hours between exercise and the alcoholic's established bedtime. Of course, exercise is also a fun, alcohol-free activity that can be enjoyed as a couple.

5. *Spend time during the day interacting with other people.* The stimulation of interacting with other people during the day has the positive effect of helping sleep. Help the alcoholic and his or her partner plan activities with other people.

6. *Establish a bedtime routine.* Help the alcoholic and his or her partner learn how to prepare for bedtime. Behaviors such as putting on pajamas, brushing teeth, reading a book, meditating, listening to music, or watching television signal to the body that sleep is to come. Of course, consistency is important in establishing a routine.

7. *If you cannot sleep, get up and do something useful.* Worrying about not sleeping can further exacerbate a disrupted sleep cycle. Help the alcoholic plan what he or she will do if sleep does not occur within 30 minutes of going to bed. For instance, behaviors such as reading a book, writing a letter, or listening to music can be a relaxing backup plan for sleepless nights.

8. *Always get up at your usual time, even if you have had a sleepless night.* Staying in bed to catch up on sleep in the morning and taking naps in the middle of the day add to an alcoholic's disrupted sleep pattern. Encourage the alcoholic to get up even after a sleepless night, and to maintain his or her established bedtime and waking time.

Exercises

1. Explore each of these guidelines with clients and assess their sleep problems and areas for improvement.

2. Have clients keep a "sleep diary" in which they record the number of hours they slept and the quality of their sleep. In addition, the clients may record the chain of events that preceded any sleep difficulties and may find a modified Drinking Chain to be helpful.

3. Explore any negative thoughts (e.g., "I never sleep well," or, "I did not sleep well this week and I am never going to catch up on my sleep").

Help clients challenge these thoughts and counter them with more rational, adaptive thoughts.

4. Encourage the couple to develop a sleep routine that works best for both of them.

WORK AND SOBRIETY

Work experiences in the early stages of sobriety may change for the better or for the worse. Alcoholics may find a new enthusiasm for their jobs that did not exist when drinking was a central factor in their lives. Some alcoholics may have worked while inebriated, and may now be experiencing a sense of clarity and increased ability to concentrate while working. With these positive changes, recovering alcoholics may feel they are accomplishing much more than they have in the past. This success may, in turn, provide the alcoholic with a positive reward loop: stop drinking, accomplish more at work, feel a renewed sense of self, and feel less of a desire to drink.

Other alcoholics may realize, once they have become sober, that they have been investing too much energy on their job and have neglected other areas of their lives. Or, they may realize that their job is not fulfilling and a change of career may be in order.

Additionally, there are many instances in which work-related difficulties contributed to the alcoholic's seeking treatment. If this is the case, the alcoholic may feel either gratitude toward, or contempt for, supervisors and coworkers depending on the level of support he or she receives upon returning to work. The issue of encountering coworkers with whom the client used to drink (outside of or even during work) also needs to be raised and discussed. Having to go to work every day and deal with pressure from old "drinking buddies" is considered a high-risk situation, and extra time should be spent exploring coping strategies to deal with such circumstances.

It is important to help the alcoholic plan ahead for the variety of reactions he or she may receive from supervisors and coworkers. Of course, difficulty on the job and unsupportive reactions from staff can trigger a relapse. Having a clear plan of action following a particularly difficult day is the alcoholic's best defense against a return to drinking behavior.

Exercises

The following exercises may be helpful in assessing work-related difficulties and addressing the client's concerns.

1. Begin by having the client describe his or her job, including the responsibilities, environment, coworkers, supervisor, wages, fringe/health benefits, promotions, rewards, and drawbacks.

2. Ask about how drinking has affected any of the above areas and how being abstinent has, or will have, an impact.

3. If either the client or the partner is concerned about the amount of time spent at work, discuss this issue and explore ways that the couple can negotiate getting both their needs met. Often, the client simply needs to learn better time management techniques, assertiveness skills for turning down work (as appropriate), or tips on delegating tasks. If the therapist has the expertise to teach these skills, it may be worthwhile spending time on this issue; otherwise, make sure the client has appropriate referrals.

4. If the client is concerned about conflict at work, help him or her problem solve, referring to the communication skills taught earlier in treatment. Clear expression of feelings (and thoughts), perception checks, and reflective listening are skills that can be as helpful at work, as at home.

5. If one of the client's concerns is having to deal with coworkers who are drinkers (or other substance abusers), reminding the client of the drink refusal skills may be helpful. Role playing a number of possible situations the client may encounters can help him or her build confidence in handling these situations if they should occur. It also may be helpful to discuss how the client can share with his or her coworkers about no longer drinking and being in treatment, if this would have beneficial effects.

6. If career counseling is in order, the therapist may address this need or make appropriate referrals. Becoming sober often leads to a reevaluation of the client's whole lifestyle, including work. Although it may be scary, job changes are often an important step to help a client remain abstinent.

Unemployment

One issue yet to be discussed is that of unemployment. Very often, as a result of excessive drinking, the client has lost his or her job or has changed jobs frequently. Unemployment is a great source of distress and financial insecurity and leads to decreased self-esteem. Helping the client locate appropriate resources (e.g., community agencies, credit counselor) for finding work and getting out of financial trouble can be a critical role for the therapist. It is very common for clients to complete an alcoholism treatment program successfully and then relapse because of overwhelming financial concerns and the devaluing experience of being unemployed. The client can be encouraged to use many of the skills taught earlier in the program to work through the difficulties of unemployment. For example, the alternative thoughts exercise can be helpful to counter negative self-statements that may hinder the client from seeking employment; the role-playing technique can be used to practice interviewing for a job; and the goal-setting process can be used to find employment and take care of financial problems.

EXERCISE AND SOBRIETY

A regular exercise program is very important in overall good health and has the added benefit of enhancing sobriety. Starting a regular exercise program can lead to improved physical and mental health, increased energy, more restful sleep, enhanced self-esteem, and may even lead to a longer, more satisfying life (Geller, 1991a).

The added benefit for people in recovery from alcoholism is that exercise is a way to feel good without alcohol. Exercise has been called the "natural high" because it stimulates the production of endorphins, which are the body's own natural chemicals that make people feel good. Alcohol is a substance that suppresses normal endorphin production. Thus, for most people who quit drinking and begin an exercise program, they may expect to experience an increase in endorphin production and very positive physical changes.

An important first step before beginning an exercise program is to consult a physician and have a medical checkup. Months or years of drinking and/or inactivity can lead to various health problems that may need to be addressed prior to beginning any exercise program. The second step is to keep in mind two key principles as far as exercise is concerned: moderation and gradual progression. It is important for the person in early recovery to start out slowly and make exercise an enjoyable experience. Moderation is also important because many alcoholics, who are used to the "I want to feel better NOW" philosophy and are just learning the benefit of "delayed gratification," tend to jump into a rigorous program that they then give up after a few weeks. Thus, starting slowly, building up strength and endurance gradually, and practicing moderation will help ensure success and continuation in an exercise program.

Exercises

The following exercises may help clients get started on a healthy exercise plan. Remind clients to consult a physician prior to beginning any exercise program.

1. Have the clients generate a list of exercise activities that they find enjoyable and to which they are well suited. Pay particular attention to those activities that the couple enjoys doing together.

2. Once the clients have chosen an activity or sport, help them stick with it by exploring the automatic thoughts and behaviors that have led to cessation of exercise in the past (e.g., "I am too tired," "I do not have time").

3. Have the clients counter their automatic thoughts and formulate new, alternative thoughts. For example, if the automatic thought is, "I'm too tired to go to the gym tonight," the alternative thought might be, "I'm tired now, but I know that I always feel better once I get to the gym."

4. Next, have the clients determine how many times a week they are willing to engage in the activity and for how long. Help them choose realistic goals, starting out slowly.

5. Explore with both clients what the best kind of support is for them and how they can receive this from each other or from friends/family.

6. Finally, the therapist can discuss with the clients how he or she will support them and how he or she will follow up with them on this goal.

7. Additional issues to explore with your clients that may help them get started and increase their commitments to exercising include the following:

- What exercise have they done in the past?
- When (times of day and days) did they do the exercise?
- How did they feel while exercising and after exercising?
- What benefits did they get from exercising at that time?
- What made them quit (paying particular attention to the maladaptive thoughts)?
- What are their current concerns and expectations about how to make exercise become a regular part of their lives?

Between 30% and 70% of the people who begin exercise programs drop out within the first 3 months. Steps 2 through 5 are critical if the clients are to continue with an exercise program. Using alternative thoughts to counter the well-rehearsed voice that says, "I don't feel like exercising tonight," "It's too cold out," or, "I'll go tomorrow" can help the clients stay on track with their exercise goals. In addition, choosing enjoyable activities in which to participate is a key element to a successful exercise program.

A further point to raise with clients is that decreased heart and lung capacity typically is the result of heavy drinking over a long period of time (Geller, 1991a). In order to improve these functions, aerobic activity (activities that increase heart rate when performed continuously) is essential. Of all the aerobic activities, the five most popular are walking, running, swimming, bicycling, and aerobic dancing. Help the client determine which of these is the most suitable and potentially enjoyable to him or her. Again, remind the eager clients to begin gradually, exercise simply and with moderate intensity (e.g. walk 15–20 minutes three times a week). Intensity and frequency can be gradually increased as strength and endurance improves.

SMOKING CESSATION AND SOBRIETY

Many alcoholics in recovery find that they would like to quit smoking as well. The feeling of satisfaction and triumph that may come from abstaining from alcohol may be one reason to give up cigarettes.

Nicotine is a psychoactive drug that falls into the same category as amphetamines and cocaine, all of which are stimulants. "The amount of nicotine that is contained in a single cigarette can raise blood pressure and increase heart and breathing rates," (Geller, 1991a, p. 326). Nicotine also increases alertness, reduces irritability and anxiety, and reduces appetite. With all of these reinforcing effects, as well as the socially acceptable manner in which smoking occurs, it is no wonder it is difficult to give up smoking. The dangers of smoking, however, far outweigh the benefits. Some common physical dangers include heart attacks, coronary artery disease, chronic lung disease (emphysema and bronchitis), and cancers of the lung, mouth, larynx, esophagus, throat, bladder, and pancreas (Palfai & Jankiewicz, 1991).

Clients may ask when is the best time to quit smoking. Some may have heard that it is best not to try to stop smoking during the first year of sobriety from alcohol. However, there is no evidence to indicate that this is so. The best time to quit may very well be as soon as possible!

There are both physical and psychological symptoms that the client may experience when he or she decides to quit smoking. Physical withdrawal from nicotine usually lasts from 3 to 5 days. The symptoms include irritability, poor concentration, sleep disturbance, fatigue, and/or headaches. Psychological withdrawal in most instances may last a longer period of time because the smoker has firmly established rituals around smoking that have been practiced routinely 20 times a day.

If a client decides that quitting smoking would increase his or her chances of remaining abstinent (because smoking is a trigger for drinking or the targeted behavior), you can use the same strategies described in this book to help the client quit smoking. For example, the Target Behavior Chart and use of alternative thoughts, role play, relaxation techniques, and enhancement of support networks can all be applied to accomplish the goal of quitting smoking.

Smoking Cessation Tips

Additional tips, which are recommended by Geller (1991a, pp. 330–334), include the following.

1. Throw away all cigarettes and other cigarette-related supplies, such as lighters, stubs, and ashtrays, in home and office.
2. Avoid and/or change routines that are associated with smoking. Change the behaviors directly associated with smoking, such as hanging around at the table after dinner or taking a coffee/smoke break. Replace those behaviors with new ones.
3. Drink six to eight glasses of water a day. Water will help flush out the toxins of the cigarettes and may help to fill the void left by quitting smoking.
4. Tell others about quitting. Family, friends, and coworkers can be great sources of support and encouragement.
5. Plan enough activities to fill the days and evenings. Make sure the client has a plan of activities to do instead of hanging around smoking.
6. Exercise regularly. Now is a good time to review the exercise program that clients may have talked about. Exercise is both a calming and an invigorating experience.
7. Avoid friends and others who smoke. The temptation to smoke with friends and others who are smoking will be great, especially in the first weeks and months of quitting. Have your clients plan activities with nonsmoking friends to get a sense of how others interact without cigarettes.
8. Eat nutritional meals. A balanced diet will give clients a sense of good health as well as help restore the body that has been exposed to nicotine for so long.

Smoking is one of the hardest addictions to conquer. Referrals to outside smoking cessation programs and/or support groups may be appropriate. Additionally, there are many great resources (books, tapes, videos, and research articles) that address tobacco addiction extensively and may be very helpful augmentations to the recommended approach.

RELAXATION AND SOBRIETY

Alcohol is one of the most common substances people use to help themselves relax. Once a client becomes abstinent from alcohol, he or she will need to learn alternative ways to relax and unwind. There are a number of specific relaxation techniques that are helpful in decreasing tension in daily life. Below is a relaxation technique that you can use with your clients in the office to teach them how to relax. The clients can practice these techniques as homework assignments or whenever they need to reduce tension. Additional suggestions and variations of relaxation techniques are included at the end.

The relaxation technique outlined below has been adapted from Goldfried and Davison (1976). The exercise takes about 20 minutes and can improve clients' ability to cope with stress and tension in their lives, as well as help them feel more energized and alert throughout the day. Emphasize that relaxation is a new skill and it is important to practice the skill in order to get the maximum benefit.

Begin by asking the clients on a scale of 0 to 10 (10 being highest) how they would rate their level of tension. Next, explain to the clients that the purpose of the exercise is to help them experience the contrast between feeling tense and feeling relaxed, with the idea that as they become more aware of these different states, they can learn to focus more on the relaxation sensations and less on the tension. Also explain that to achieve this goal, you will lead them through a process of tensing and relaxing different parts of their bodies. Before beginning, ask if they have any concerns about participating in this exercise or need more information before you move on.

When clients are ready, have them settle back as comfortably as they can and close their eyes. If they are initially uncomfortable closing their eyes, invite them to look down at their hands or at the floor. Then, have them pay attention to their breathing, until their breath comes slowly and easily. Next, have them imagine themselves in a favorite, safe, and soothing place—pausing to give them enough time to get there. Proceed by following the narrative below, making sure to pause frequently and allow the clients plenty of time to experience the sensations.

Sample Narrative

"We are going to begin now by having you focus on different parts of your body, starting with your left hand. So bring all of your attention to your left hand (*pause*), allowing any distracting thoughts or feelings to just drift on by. Notice any tingling or tightness that might be present. Now, I want you to clench your left fist tightly and feel the tension in your hand and forearm . . . that's it, hold it . . . , just a little bit more . . . , and RELAX. That's it, just allow all of the tension to drain away and feel the muscles relax (*pause*). Notice the contrast between the tension and relaxation and allow the feelings of relaxation to begin to flow through you (*pause*). And BREATHE . . . that's it, feel your breath come smoothly and easily.

"Now, we are going to move up your arm to your forearm. Again, notice any tension or tightness that is present (*pause*). Okay, now tighten your muscles in your forearm as tight as you can . . . that's it, hold it . . . , just a little bit more . . . , and LET GO. That's it, just allow all of the tension to drain away, out through your fingertips and feel all of your muscles RELAX (*pause*). Once again, notice the contrast between the tension and relaxation, focusing now on the feelings of relaxation in your left hand and forearm (*pause*). And BREATHE. . . ."

Follow this same procedure, moving to the upper left arm, then the right hand, right forearm, and right upper arm. Then, move on to the shoulders, having the clients begin by shrugging their shoulders, bringing both shoulders up towards their ears, tightening and holding, then letting go and relaxing the muscles.

Next, move to the neck, and have the clients press their heads back against the surface on which they are resting, until they can feel the tension. Hold the tension, once again tightening, holding, and finally letting go, "letting your head rest comfortably and enjoying the contrast between the tension you created and the relaxation you feel now." Next, bring their focus to the front of their necks, having them bury their chins into their chests, following the same procedure of tightening and relaxing. Move on to the face, instructing the clients to tighten all their facial muscles, by scrunching up their faces, closing their eyes even tighter, holding, tightening, holding, and finally . . . letting go.

You can move through the rest of the body, as time allows. The chest, abdomen, buttocks, upper right leg, lower right leg (calf), right foot, upper left leg, lower left leg, and left foot. Remember to pause frequently and remind them to breathe. When you've gone as far as time allows, gently complete the exercise (e.g., "Allow yourselves to slowly come back into the room, and when you feel ready, open your eyes and look into your hands"). Take another rating of the clients' level of tension at this point (from 0 to 10) and compare this rating with the rating at the beginning of the exercise. Allow enough time to have the clients give feedback and describe how the exercise went for each of them.

Suggestions and Variations

1. Of course, the therapist can change the order of the exercise and begin with the feet instead of the hands, play music, dim the lights, and/or record the exercise so that the clients may take the tape home with them.

2. Another relaxation technique is a guided imagery exercise in which the clients simply sit back, close their eyes, focus on their breathing,

and imagine a pleasant scene—all with the purpose of helping the clients calm down and relax.

3. It is important that the clients *practice* these exercises. It is possible that, if they practice regularly (a few times per week), eventually, just by closing their eyes and imagining their favorite place, they will be able to decrease their pulse rate and relax their bodies. Have them take their pulse before and after the exercise to illustrate this point.

4. Setting aside quiet time, when they won't be interrupted, to practice the exercise is very important.

5. Let the clients know that it is better not to drink caffeine or have a cigarette just before the exercise, so that they aren't having to fight against the chemical stimulants, in addition to their own natural tension.

TERMINATION PHASE

CHAPTER 9

Phase V:
End of Treatment

OVERVIEW

Discussion of Termination
Creating Individualized Long-Term Recovery Plans
Closure
   ♦ Feedback, Acknowledgments, and Goodbyes
   ♦ Certificate of Completion

Materials Needed:
   ♦ Session Notes for Review
   ♦ Two Recovery Plans (Form 11)
   ♦ Certificate of Completion (Form 12)
   ♦ Pencils and Clipboards

Recommended number of sessions: 2

Goals: 1. Discuss termination of treatment.
*   2. Create a long-term Recovery Plan.*
*   3. Conclude therapy successfully.*

The Termination Phase of therapy is designed to allow time for clients to discuss their thoughts and feelings about concluding therapy and to make plans for long-term recovery. The clients need time to acknowledge their successes, as well as time to discuss any fears they have about ending the therapeutic relationship. In addition, we introduce a Recovery Plan which is designed to help clients make concrete plans for continuing to work on their abstinence and focus on issues that will enhance their sobriety. To close, we suggest presenting clients with a certificate of completion which is introduced at the end of this chapter.

DISCUSSION OF TERMINATION

Introduce the topic of termination of therapy and summarize the previous Relapse Prevention sessions. Acknowledge clients' successes in reaching their goals, and make note of any problem areas that still need to be addressed. Ask the clients to discuss their thoughts and feelings about the cessation of treatment.

Rationale

It is important to address concerns regarding termination of therapy as soon as they arise. Although we are suggesting these concerns be formally addressed in Session 18 (if you are following the 20-session model), they are likely to arise earlier in treatment and should be addressed accordingly. However, setting aside time specifically to discuss the clients' feelings and thoughts, especially any maladaptive thoughts (e.g., "treatment is over, so maybe I can drink now") about the cessation of treatment is critical. The purpose of this discussion is that, as Beck and his colleagues state, "when the conclusion of therapy is handled well, the patient is more likely to consolidate gains and to generalize strategies for handling future problems" (Beck et al., 1979, p. 317).

1. Consolidating gains and generalizing learned skills to everyday life is one of the main goals of the treatment. Thus, when clients express maladaptive thoughts that may impede the achievement of this goal (e.g., "I can't do this on my own" or "I know I'm going to relapse without therapy"), the thoughts must be addressed and challenged. Additionally, it is important to remind the couple that they have learned more effective ways to support themselves and each other during this treatment that they can count on when therapy ends.

2. Completing treatment may be the first accomplishment the client(s) have achieved in a long time, because drinking often interferes with the successful attainment of goals. Thus, it is important to reinforce this positive action. Furthermore, this may be the first activity *the couple* has seen through, from beginning to end, in a long time and the joint accomplishment should be reinforced.

Procedure

Step 1. Ask clients to share what they have learned about themselves, about each other, and about staying abstinent from alcohol and the target behavior.

Step 2. Discuss the clients' successes and problem areas throughout the program thus far, and explain that, by identifying the remaining problem areas, there is still time to decide on a plan of action to work on those issues when the program ends. Briefly explain that the next two sessions will be spent creating a Recovery Plan and saying good-bye.

Step 3. Continue to be aware of the clients' reactions to the cessation of therapy and ask them about their thoughts and feelings. Ask about how they will spend their free time without the structure and routine of this program. If appropriate, remind clients that they are not "quitting," that the treatment was designed as a 20-session program that they have successfully completed. It is just the beginning of their recovery process, and they are beginning that process with a whole new array of coping strategies and resources.

Step 4. If clients are expressing negative thoughts that may interfere with recovery, overtly address these thoughts as you have done with other problematic thoughts, having clients counter negative thoughts and formulate adaptive, rationale alternative thoughts (refer to the section on Cognitive Coping Skills in Chapter 6). For example:

Negative thought:	"I can't stay sober on my own without therapy."
Feeling:	Fear
Alternative thoughts:	"I've learned a lot of skills to use at home." "I've been on my own every other week when we haven't had a session." "I have my wife and friends to help me out."
Feeling:	Less fear, relief, hope

As Beck and colleagues (1979, 1993) point out, having the clients answer their own concerns and respond to their own dysfunctional thoughts reinforces their ability to use the skills they have learned and increases their sense of confidence in generalizing these skills.

Step 5. Clients may also take this time to express their appreciation for the therapy and the gains they have made. Termination of therapy is not always a fearful time for clients; for many, it is a time to celebrate their accomplishments. Of course, celebrating without drinking may be another issue to discuss!

Exercises

1. Have clients discuss with each other their successes and areas for improvement.

2. Have clients discuss with each other how they feel about ending treatment and any concerns they have for each other. Have them bring feedback to the next session.

3. Have clients discuss and write down their ideas about how they plan on maintaining abstinence once treatment ends (e.g., attend AA, continue therapy, practice specific skills). Have them bring the written plans to the next session.

CREATING INDIVIDUALIZED LONG-TERM RECOVERY PLANS

In this section, we describe the collaborative development of a long-term Recovery Plan. The purposes of the Recovery Plan (Form 11) are (1) to give the clients something tangible to take with them that identifies what they have learned during the program, (2) to help them make concrete plans for continuing recovery, and (3) to write down resources/referrals for handling ongoing concerns and/or where to get help if they lapse or relapse.

Rationale

Researchers and clinicians have identified a variety of strategies for helping the alcoholic to plan ahead for high-risk situations and to prevent relapse, including Marlatt and Gordon's (1985) Relapse Road Maps, Monti et al.'s (1989) Seemingly Irrelevant Decisions Reminder Sheet and Planning for Emergencies Reminder Sheet (pp. 223–224), and Gorski's (1989) Addictive Self and Sober Self worksheets (pp. 55–57). The Recovery Plan is a two-page worksheet designed with the same purposes in mind, which may be used independently or in conjunction with any of these other plans.

Having a detailed plan of action to maintain abstinence and continue working on persistent problem areas is an essential treatment component. Being able to handle emergencies, high-risk situations, and unplanned life events will be critical skills for the clients to attain in order to maintain abstinence. Thus, if the clients are given the opportunity to prepare a plan of action that will help them cope with unexpected occurrences and remind them of the skills learned in the program, their chances of remaining abstinent will be increased.

Procedure

Step 1. Begin this treatment component by reviewing the many skills that the clients have learned throughout the program, first eliciting as many as possible from the clients (e.g., drink/target behavior refusal, communication skills, relaxation), and then filling in those they have omitted. Ask the clients to share with each other how they plan to implement these skills when the program is complete.

Step 2. Challenge the clients to think of all the different aspects of their lives (e.g., home, work, school, relationship with each other, relationship with their children) and how they can implement or continue implementing these skills in these areas. Explain that applying the coping and communication skills to their daily lives is crucial for ongoing, successful abstinence.

Step 3. Explain the purpose of a Recovery Plan (Form 11) and give the clients a chance to express how this device might be helpful to them.

Step 4. Go back over the in-session and at-home exercises, noting ones that have been especially helpful. Have clients write down what they have learned during the program in Section I of the Recovery Plan (see Figure 9.1). Have them give each other feedback regarding changes they have noticed in each other.

Step 5. Give the clients feedback regarding anything else that you think they learned or gained during treatment. Allow them time to include this on the Recovery Plan.

Step 6. Discuss with both clients what they want to continue working on when the program ends, in order to maintain their abstinence and continue with their personal growth. (They may refer to their Action Plans, as needed.)

Step 7. Have the clients brainstorm together strategies for dealing with these remaining concerns and provide feedback as necessary.

Step 8. After completing Steps 6 and 7 above, ask the clients to record on their Recovery Plans, in Section II, those problems they are willing to work on and how they plan on doing so (see Figure 9.1). It is important that clients include only those problems they are really willing to work toward addressing at this point in time. Have clients be realistic in their goals so as to increase chances of success.

I. WHAT I LEARNED IN THE PROGRAM:

♦ I learned to notice what is happening around me and what makes me want to drink.

♦ I learned how important it is for me to tell my partner when her behaviors are supportive of my sobriety.

(Leave space for the clients to add feedback from the therapist about changes he or she observed in the clients during the program.)

II. WHAT I WILL CONTINUE TO WORK ON AND HOW I WILL WORK ON IT (BE SPECIFIC):

♦ I will continue to work on my sobriety by attending 3 AA meetings per week.

♦ I will continue to work on my sobriety by using the relaxation exercise twice a week.

♦ I will work on quitting smoking by joining a smoking cessation program by January 10th.

III. HIGH-RISK SITUATIONS AND PLANS TO COPE:

Feb. 15:   Carla's wedding: Remind friends beforehand that I'm no longer drinking.

March: Tax time: Do extra relaxation exercises, exercise, and attend more AA meetings.

April: Business trip: Tell my work partner about my abstinence before the trip and make plans to call my partner during the trip for additional support.

June 12:   Anniversary of Father's death: Go to church, talk to family.

August 2:   One year anniversary of sobriety: Go to extra AA meetings, talk to friends, see therapist for a booster session.

IV. SUPPORT RESOURCES I WILL USE INCLUDE:

♦ I will call my sister, Sharon, when I feel like drinking. Her phone number is 555-0000.

♦ I will go for a walk around the block when I get angry or anxious.

♦ I will call my friend Bill when I am at a social gathering and feel uncomfortable. His phone numbers are 555-1111 (h) and 555-2222 (w).

♦ I will join the local gym and start exercising by February 1st.

♦ I will save $50/month so that we can get away on the weekends
to alleviate stress.

V. HOW MY PARTNER WILL SUPPORT ME:

(Completed by partner): I will support you, Michael, by continuing
to tell you how pleased I am about your sobriety. I will also continue
to abstain from alcohol.

VI. OTHER HELPFUL REMINDERS:

I remember a great phrase from AA: HALT—whenever I'm I Iungry,
Angry, Lonely, or Tired—is a high-risk situation. When I am in a difficult situation, I can use cognitive coping skills, especially when
there is nothing I can do to change the situation.

FIGURE 9.1. Sample Recovery Plan.

Step 9. In Section III, have clients write down any high-risk situations they anticipate arising in the next 6 months (e.g., daughter's wedding, business trip, change of income, anniversary of sobriety) and how they plan to cope with each situation. Ask them to be as specific as possible in their plans.

Step 10. In Section IV, clients are to record the list of resources they are willing to tap when necessary, including AA, Al-Anon, friends, therapy, taking vacations, going to church, and so forth. (They may refer to earlier Support Network, Form 9). The purpose of rewriting these resources on their Recovery Plans is to have everything on one sheet so as to be easily accessible.

Step 11. Ask the clients to fill in Section V on each other's Recovery Plan. This should include statements about how they will continue to support one another in their recovery. It may be helpful to have the couple take some time to discuss the most effective ways they can support each other and the ineffective ways they interact with each other. A useful formula for this discussion, to be repeated as many times as necessary, is as follows:

Alcoholic Client to Partner:

"I feel supported by you when you _____ [specific behavior]."

"I do not feel supported by you when _____ [specific behavior]."

Partner to Alcoholic Client:

"I feel supported by you when you _____ [specific behavior]."

"I do not feel supported by you when _____ [specific behavior]."

For example:

Alcoholic to Partner:

"I feel supported when you compliment me on the changes I've made so far. I do not feel supported when you ask me if I'm going to AA meetings."

Partner to Alcoholic (target behavior: abstaining from sweets):

"I feel supported when you don't eat ice cream in front of me. I do not feel supported when you ask me how much weight I've lost."

Step 12. The last section, Section VI, is for clients to add any other "helpful hints" they have found to be of value in maintaining abstinence. This may be something that stood out for clients during treatment or, perhaps, something important heard at an AA meeting.

Step 13. Discuss with clients how they will use their Recovery Plans (e.g., how often they will look at them, where they will keep them, when they will update them). Encourage clients to review the Recovery Plans regularly in order to be reminded of the skills they possess to cope with difficult situations and to reinforce the positive changes made in their lives.

Exercises

1. If clients are unable to complete the Recovery Plans in one session (which will most likely be the case), have clients complete them at home and bring them to the next session.

2. Have clients give each other input for their Recovery Plans.

3. Have clients continue to write down or discuss with each other thoughts related to the completion of the program for discussion in the last session.

4. Have the couple plan a pleasant event to celebrate their success in completing the program.

CLOSURE

Feedback, Acknowledgments, and Goodbyes

Take the opportunity to (1) go over any last thoughts or feelings regarding treatment closure, (2) ask clients for feedback about the overall program, (3) acknowledge the clients for their successes and give them feedback on their progress throughout the program, (4) ask the clients to acknowledge each other, and (5) make agreements about future contact with the clients (e.g., 3-, 6-, or 12-month follow-ups).

Certificates of Completion

Each client is given a "Certificate of Completion" during the final session of treatment (see Form 12). The certificate serves as a pleasant reminder of all the hard work the clients accomplished during the program. Some clients may choose to frame their certificate and display it as a daily reminder of their sobriety.

Case Illustration: Ending Treatment

Mike and Beth are excited to be completing the program, as well as a little fearful to be "on their own." Both partners have done well in treatment. Mike relapsed twice during the 5-month program and Beth relapsed on caffeine six times. (It took awhile in the beginning for Beth to take her commitment seriously and try hard to abstain from caffeine; however, when she began to see the parallels between her thinking and behavior and Mike's, especially after his first relapse, she recommitted to the goal.) Mike's second relapse resulted in another DUI and he has since given up the idea that he can drink "socially" or "moderately."

Mike developed a strong Recovery Plan including attending AA meetings, continuing to work out at a local gym, and spending time with friends and family (he has made a couple of new, sober friends since the program began). Beth also developed a strong Recovery Plan for herself including going back to school one night a week, spending time with friends, and making more time for pleasant events with Mike.

The couple do not plan on continuing in therapy on an ongoing basis, but agree to continue practicing the many skills they learned in treatment. In particular, the couple find the communication skills and drink refusal skills helpful. At the conclusion of treatment, both partners are actively using alternative cognitive and behavioral coping strategies. Beth is particularly strong at countering her automatic thoughts regarding *needing* or *deserving* a cup of coffee. Mike, however, has a more difficult time grasping the concept of countering thoughts and actively engages more behavioral strategies, such as leaving a situation where he is tempted to drink, talking to Beth about his cravings, and using relaxation techniques regularly. He has also made some changes in his work environment that have resulted in decreased stress. His relationship with Beth has improved dramatically as they both engage in more functional communication skills, spend more time doing "pleasant events" with each other, and enjoy a more satisfying and intimate sexual relationship.

The couple are pleased with their Certificates of Completion and Mike reports that this was the first "project" he has completed since he started drinking heavily 3 years ago.

APPENDICES

Suggested Meeting Schedule for 20-Session Therapy Model

I. MEET TWO TIMES PER WEEK FOR 6 WEEKS:

Session 1: Program logistics; building rapport; confidentiality; history taking.

Session 2: Treatment expectations; discussion of treatment goals.

Session 3: Conclude intake/assessment; behavioral contracting.

Session 4: Introduce self-monitoring charts—Drinking Chain I (DCI) and Target Behavior Chart I (TBCI); introduce Communication Skills: Level I.

Session 5: Review of DCI and TBCI; communication skills training; introduce pleasant events.

Session 6: Review of DCI and TBCI; communication skills training; follow up on pleasant events.

Session 7: Review of DCI and TBCI; introduce Communication Skills: Level II; follow up on pleasant events.

Session 8: Introduce new charts, Drinking Chain II (DCII) and Target Behavior Chart II (TBCII); follow up on pleasant events; communication skills training.

Session 9: Review of DCII and TBCII; follow up on pleasant events; introduce cognitive and behavioral coping skills training.

Session 10: Review of DCII and TBCII; follow up on pleasant events; cognitive and behavioral coping skills training.

Session 11: Review of DCII and TBCII; cognitive and behavioral coping skills training; introduce drink/target behavior refusal training; introduce Communication Skills: Level III.

Session 12: Review of DCII and TBCII; cognitive and behavioral coping skills training; follow up on drink/target behavioral refusal training; termination of Acute Phase of Treatment.

II. MEET ONCE A WEEK FOR 3 WEEKS:

Session 13: Evaluate progress and assess abstinence; prioritize recovery needs and introduce Options.

Session 14: Explore support network; create Action Plan.

Session 15: Implement Action Plan interventions; continue working on enhancing support network.

III. MEET ONCE EVERY OTHER WEEK FOR 8 WEEKS:

Session 16: Implement Action Plan interventions; review cognitive and behavioral coping skills, as necessary; review communication skills, as necessary; review support network issues, as necessary.

Session 17: Same as in Session 16.

Session 18: Same as in Session 16.

Session 19: Discuss termination; create individualized long-term Recovery Plans.

IV. SKIP 2 WEEKS AND MEET FOR THE LAST TIME:

Session 20: Complete Recovery Plans; closure; Certificate of Completion.

Exploring Triggers

I. INTRODUCTION

The trigger column on the Drinking Chain I and Target Behavior Chart I may be the most difficult for the clients to understand and complete. However, this column is a critical aspect of both the Drinking Chain and the Target Behavior Chart.

The purpose of identifying the trigger is to help clients become more aware of what it is that precedes their episodes of drinking or engaging in the target behavior. Most people begin to believe that they have no control over using a substance and that it "just happens." We are teaching the alcoholics that if the stimuli that initiate their drinking episodes can be identified, then they will stand a better chance of consciously saying "no," and deciding on another behavior. We are teaching the partner a similar task, that is, to learn to identify the stimuli that initiate engagement in the target behavior. This ability will give the partner the opportunity to decide whether to engage in the target behavior or to choose another behavior.

An added benefit of identifying the trigger is to help clients discover those situations that are "high risk." For example, if a client's trigger is a combination of the thought about paying bills and a feeling of anxiousness, then it is clear that handling finances is a high-risk situation for the client. Finding alternative thoughts to manage this situation, as well as finding alternative coping strategies to address the anxiety are important treatment interventions.

II. GENERAL GUIDELINES

1. Make sure that the client identifies the situation as clearly as possible.
2. Ask the client: "What happened?"; or, "What did you notice just before you decided to drink?"; or, "What did you tell yourself right before you decided to drink?" (Of course, you can use the same strategy with the partner).
3. If the client cannot answer, "walk through" the situation he or she wrote down and have him or her "make up" what happened. Eventually, as he or she becomes more aware about the components of the event, triggers will be easily identified.
4. Offer suggestions if the client cannot come up with the trigger.
5. Another helpful approach to elicit triggers for those who cannot remember is to ask: "What was the straw that broke the camel's back?"; or, "What was the thing that flipped the switch and made you drink (or engage in target behavior)?" People often respond to these analogies more readily.
6. Elicit the help of the partner; he or she might be able to fill in the missing pieces of what actually happened.

III. SAMPLE NARRATIVE

THERAPIST: You said that you were at home watching television with your wife and your son. Earlier in the evening you had been paying bills and you were feeling frustrated about your financial situation. Is this correct?

CLIENT: Yes, and it was about 9:00 P.M..

THERAPIST: What happened right before you decided that you wanted a beer?

CLIENT: I don't know. I was just watching television.

THERAPIST: Do you remember if there was a commercial or something happening on the show that made you think of drinking?

CLIENT: No, I don't think so.

THERAPIST (*to partner*): Do you recall anything that might have triggered his desire to drink?

FEMALE CLIENT: Well, our son's friend came over and they were talking about going out. Was that around the same time?

CLIENT: Oh yeah. You're right. Hmmm. . . . Yeah, I remember now thinking about how I owe Steve's [son's friend] dad $50 for some tickets.

THERAPIST: And, you were already feeling frustrated about your finances. Do you think this might have been the trigger—thinking about how you were going to pay him and feeling worried?

CLIENT: Well, yeah, I suppose so. As soon as I saw Steve, I got up and went to the refrigerator. I think I was trying to avoid seeing Steve and thinking about the money I owe his dad.

THERAPIST: Are you beginning to see how important it is to walk through the situation? There was more happening than you thought. We now know that when you are frustrated and anxious about money you are in a high-risk situation. A high-risk situation like this one leads you to think about and want a drink.

IV. CONCLUSIONS

Being able to identify the trigger to a drinking episode, or an episode where the partner engages in the target behavior, is a critical point in the recovery process. Once the client is able to identify a trigger, he or she is more likely to utilize an alternative coping strategy. This is a difficult step for most clients because they often feel like "it just happened" and they had no control over the incident. Once they realize that it did not "just happen," that there was indeed a trigger, they have to take responsibility for intervening in order to remain abstinent. The therapist helps the client identify the trigger and explore alternative strategies for coping with the trigger.

Compliance Enhancers

I. INTRODUCTION

In behavior therapy, compliance with out-of-session exercises is quite frequently a problem and this treatment program offers no exception. Some clients may fail to see the point of doing out-of-session assignments regardless of the therapist's stated purpose. However, the therapist is in a position to reinforce the fact that, without completion of the exercises, treatment cannot progress.

II. GENERAL GUIDELINES

Below are a number of guidelines helpful in fostering compliance with out-of-session assignments. Review these guidelines at the beginning of treatment and again as noncompliance arises in treatment.

1. Learn the client's expectations about treatment. Make sure that the client's expectations match the treatment goals.
2. In the early stages of treatment, give easy assignments that are likely to be completed. This affords opportunities for the therapist to award praise and helps establish the therapist as a reinforcing stimulus. In addition, clients begin to experience a sense of mastery. Collaborate as much as possible with clients when thinking of exercises that may be helpful.
3. Prior to giving the assignment, provide a clear rationale for its usefulness. Make sure the clients understand *why* they are doing a particular assignment.

4. Be sure that, when explaining an assignment, specific details are provided. For instance, how, when, for how long, and in what circumstances the assignment is to be performed. *Negotiate* with the clients, as necessary.
5. Clients must believe that the assignment is useful and acceptable. Take time to elicit the clients' beliefs, fears, and expectations regarding compliance with the assignments.
6. Take time to evaluate the clients' environment carefully. Are there constraints in the clients' social or physical environment that are impeding completion of the exercise?
7. After an assignment is given, question the clients regarding their reactions to the assignment. Engage the clients in determining when and where they will complete the assignment.
8. If therapist receives blank looks or expressions of confusion, repeat the instructions and ask the clients to paraphrase their understanding of the assignment. When the client restates the assignment, both therapist and clients should acknowledge that they understand it.
9. Review with the clients that they have signed a contract to come to sessions and to complete their out-of-session exercises.
10. Ask the clients to do a practice assignment in the session so that the therapist is available to field questions that might arise when they do the main assignment.
11. A "slip" in compliance can be treated not as a failure but as an opportunity to further self-understanding. Keep in mind that the goal is to prevent the next slip from occurring.

III. SUMMARY

Some or all of the above guidelines may be useful for the therapist to enhance compliance of out-of-session work. It is important to emphasize the necessity of completing out-of-session assignments on time, as a way to stay on track and to maximize the benefits available in this treatment approach. Take time early in treatment to work through blocks and excuses for completing these exercises.

Marlatt and Gordon's (1985) Relapse Prevention Model (Abbreviated Version)

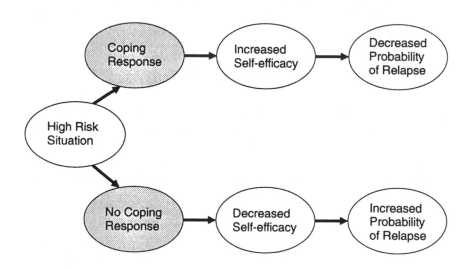

Note. Adapted from Marlatt and Gordon (1985). Copyright 1985 by The Guilford Press. Adapted by permission.

FORMS

FORM 1 DRINKING CHAIN I

Record in the spaces below each time you either drank or thought about drinking alcohol. Bring this chart with you to each therapy session.

DAY & TIME	SITUATION Where were you? What were you doing? Who were you with?	TRIGGER What happened?	DRINK OR NOT?	RESULTS & ALTERNATIVES What resulted from decision and alternative behaviors?
EXAMPLE 1: Friday 7 P.M.	Ed and Mary's house having dinner.	Ed offered me wine.	Yes	Drank four glasses (16 oz.) at Ed's. Bought bottle (32 oz.) on the way home and drank it. Argued with wife.
EXAMPLE 2: Sunday 1 P.M.	Home alone, watching the game.	Commercial for beer	No	Walked around the block during the commercials.

167

FORM 2 TARGET BEHAVIOR CHART I

Behavior to reduce or eliminate: _____

Record in the spaces below each time you either engaged in or thought about engaging in the target behavior. Bring this chart with you to each therapy session.

DAY & TIME	SITUATION Where were you? What were you doing? Who were you with?	TRIGGER What happened?	ENGAGE OR NOT?	RESULTS & ALTERNATIVES What resulted from decision and alternative behaviors?
EXAMPLE 1: Friday 6 A.M.	In kitchen getting ready for work. (target behavior: abstain from caffeine)	I was very tired and saw the coffee maker	Yes	Stopped for coffee on the way to work. Drank it at the office.
EXAMPLE 2: Monday 5 P.M.	Driving home from work. (target behavior: abstain from sugar)	Drove past the new ice cream store	No	Didn't stop for ice cream. Went home and made dinner.

FORM 3 EXERCISE RECORD

Client

SESSION	ASSIGNMENT	DATE DUE	COMPLETED
1			
2			
3			
4			
5			
6			
7			
8			
9			
10			
11			
12			

(continued)

FORM 3 *(continued)*

SESSION	ASSIGNMENT	DATE DUE	COMPLETED
13			
14			
15			
16			
17			
18			
19			
20			

FORM 4 PLEASANT EVENTS SCHEDULE

Completing this form will take you approximately 1 hour. You should plan to fill it out in a quiet place and at a time when you will not be interrupted. Read each of the 223 items and ask yourself this question:

How pleasant, enjoyable, or rewarding do I find this event?

Answer this question by rating each event on the following scale:

0—This is not pleasant (use this rating for events that are either neutral or unpleasant).

1—This is somewhat pleasant (use this rating for events that are mildly or moderately pleasant).

2—This is very pleasant (use this rating for events that are strongly or extremely pleasant).

Place your rating for each event in Column P (pleasantness).

Use the last 3 lines to add items that were not included on this list.

	P	S
1. Being in the country		
2. Wearing expensive or formal clothes and going out		
3. Making contributions to religious, charitable, or other groups		
4. Talking about sports		
5. Going to a rock concert		
6. Playing baseball or softball		
7. Planning trips or vacations		
8. Buying things for myself		
9. Being at the beach		
10. Doing art work (painting, sculpture, drawing, moviemaking, etc.)		
11. Rock climbing or mountaineering		
12. Reading the Scriptures or other sacred works		
13. Playing golf		

(continued)

FORM 4   *(continued)*

	P	S
14. Taking part in military activities		
15. Rearranging or redecorating my room or house		
16. Going to a sports event		
17. Going to the races (horse, car, boat, etc.)		
18. Reading stories, novels, poems, or plays		
19. Going to lectures or hearing speakers		
20. Thinking up or arranging a song or music		
21. Boating (canoeing, kayaking, motorboating, sailing, wind surfing, etc.)		
22. Restoring antiques, refinishing furniture, and so forth		
23. Watching TV		
24. Camping		
25. Working in politics		
26. Working on machines (cars, bikes, motorcycles, tractors, etc.)		
27. Playing cards		
28. Laughing		
29. Solving a problem, puzzle, crossword, and so forth		
30. Being at weddings, baptisms, confirmations, and so forth		
31. Having lunch with friends or associates		
32. Playing tennis		
33. Taking a shower		
34. Driving long distances		
35. Doing woodworking or carpentry		
36. Writing stories, novels, plays, or poetry		

(continued)

FORM 4 *(continued)*

	P	S
37. Riding in an airplane		
38. Exploring (hiking away from known routes, spelunking, etc.)		
39. Having a frank and open conversation		
40. Singing in a group		
41. Working at my job		
42. Going to a party		
43. Going to church functions (socials, classes, bazaars, etc.)		
44. Speaking a foreign language		
45. Going to service, civic, or social club meetings		
46. Going to a business meeting or convention		
47. Being in a sporty or expensive car		
48. Playing a musical instrument		
49. Snow skiing, snow boarding		
50. Acting		
51. Taking a nap		
52. Being with friends		
53. Canning, freezing, making preserves, and so forth		
54. Driving fast		
55. Being in a city		
56. Taking a bath		
57. Singing to myself		
58. Making food or crafts to sell or give away		
59. Playing pool or billiards		
60. Being with my children or grandchildren		

(continued)

FORM 4 *(continued)*

	P	S
61. Playing chess or checkers		
62. Doing craft work (pottery, jewelry, leather, beads, weaving, etc.)		
63. Putting on makeup, fixing my hair, and so forth		
64. Designing or drafting		
65. Visiting people who are sick, shut in, or in trouble		
66. Bowling		
67. Watching wild animals		
68. Gardening, landscaping, or doing yard work		
69. Reading essays or technical, academic, or professional literature		
70. Dancing		
71. Sitting in the sun		
72. Riding a motorcycle		
73. Just sitting and thinking		
74. Going to a fair, carnival, circus, zoo, or amusement park		
75. Talking about philosophy or religion		
76. Planning or organizing something		
77. Listening to the sounds of nature		
78. Dating		
79. Racing in a car, motorcycle, boat, and so forth		
80. Listening to the radio		
81. Having friends come to visit		
82. Playing in a sporting competition		
83. Giving gifts		
84. Going to school or government meetings, court sessions, and so forth		

(continued)

FORM 4   *(continued)*

	P	S
85. Getting massages or backrubs		
86. Watching the sky, clouds, or a storm		
87. Going on outings (to the park, a picnic, a barbecue, etc.)		
88. Playing basketball		
89. Buying something for my family		
90. Photography		
91. Giving a speech or lecture		
92. Reading maps		
93. Gathering natural objects (wild foods or fruit, rocks, driftwood, etc.)		
94. Working with computers		
95. Making a major purchase or investment (car, appliance, house, stocks, etc.)		
96. Helping someone		
97. Being in the mountains		
98. Hearing jokes		
99. Talking about my children or grandchildren		
100. Going to a revival or crusade		
101. Seeing beautiful scenery		
102. Eating good meals		
103. Improving my health (having my teeth fixed, getting new glasses, changing my diet, etc.)		
104. Wrestling or boxing		
105. Hunting or shooting		
106. Playing in a musical group		
107. Hiking		
108. Going to a museum or exhibit		

(continued)

FORM 4 *(continued)*

	P	S
109. Writing papers, essays, articles, reports, memos, and so forth		
110. Fishing		
111. Counseling someone		
112. Going to a health club, sauna bath, and so forth		
113. Learning to do something new		
114. Going out to dinner		
115. Complimenting or praising someone		
116. Thinking about people I like		
117. Being with my parents		
118. Horseback riding		
119. Protesting social, political, or environmental conditions		
120. Talking on the telephone		
121. Having daydreams		
122. Kicking leaves, sand, pebbles, and so forth		
123. Playing lawn sports (badminton, croquet, shuffleboard, horseshoes, etc.)		
124. Going to school reunions, alumni meetings, and so forth		
125. Seeing famous people		
126. Going to the movies		
127. Kissing		
128. Being alone		
129. Cooking or baking		
130. Feeling the presence of the Lord in my life		
131. Doing "odd jobs" around the house		
132. Being at a family reunion or get-together		

(continued)

FORM 4 *(continued)*

	P	S
133. Giving a party or get-together		
134. Coaching someone		
135. Going to a restaurant		
136. Seeing or smelling a flower or plant		
137. Receiving honors (civic, military, etc.)		
138. Reminiscing, talking about old times		
139. Getting up early in the morning		
140. Having peace and quiet		
141. Doing experiments or other scientific work		
142. Visiting friends		
143. Writing in a diary		
144. Playing football		
145. Being counseled		
146. Saying prayers		
147. Giving massages or backrubs		
148. Hitchhiking		
149. Meditating or doing yoga		
150. Doing favors for people		
151. Being relaxed		
152. Playing board games (Monopoly, Scrabble, etc.)		
153. Doing heavy outdoor work (cutting or chopping wood, clearing land, farm work, etc.)		
154. Reading the newspaper		
155. Snowmobiling or dune-buggy riding		
156. Being in a body-awareness, sensitivity, encounter, therapy, or "rap" group		
157. Playing ping-pong		

(continued)

FORM 4   *(continued)*

	P	S
158. Swimming		
159. Running, jogging, or doing gymnastics, fitness, or field exercises		
160. Walking barefoot		
161. Playing frisbee or catch		
162. Doing housework or laundry; cleaning things		
163. Being with my roommate		
164. Listening to music		
165. Knitting, crocheting, or doing embroidery or fancy needlework		
166. Being intimate with someone		
167. Amusing people		
168. Talking about sex		
169. Going to a barber or beautician		
170. Having house guests		
171. Being with someone I love		
172. Reading magazines		
173. Sleeping late		
174. Starting a new project		
175. Having sexual relations		
176. Having other sexual satisfactions		
177. Going to the library		
178. Playing soccer, rugby, hockey, lacrosse, and so forth		
179. Preparing a new or special food		
180. Birdwatching		
181. Shopping		

(continued)

FORM 4 *(continued)*

	P	S
182. Watching people		
183. Building or watching a fire		
184. Selling or trading something		
185. Finishing a project or task		
186. Repairing things		
187. Working with others as a team		
188. Bicycling		
189. Playing party games		
190. Writing letters, cards, or notes		
191. Talking about politics or public affairs		
192. Going to banquets, luncheons, potlucks, and so forth		
193. Talking about my hobby or special interest		
194. Smiling at people		
195. Playing in sand, a stream, the grass, and so forth		
196. Being with my husband, wife, or partner		
197. Expressing my love to someone		
198. Caring for houseplants		
199. Having coffee, tea, a coke, and so forth with friends		
200. Sewing		
201. Remembering a departed friend or loved one, visiting the cemetary		
202. Doing things with children		
203. Beachcombing		
204. Staying up late		
205. Being with my children		

(continued)

FORM 4 *(continued)*

	P	S
206. Going to auctions, garage sales, and so forth		
207. Doing volunteer work, working on community service projects		
208. Water skiing, surfing, scuba diving		
209. Defending or protecting someone, stopping fraud or abuse		
210. Hearing a good sermon		
211. Picking up a hitchhiker		
212. Winning a competition		
213. Talking about my job or school		
214. Reading cartoons, comic strips, or comic books		
215. Traveling with friends or a group		
216. Seeing old friends		
217. Teaching someone		
218. Traveling by myself		
219. Going to office parties or departmental get-togethers		
220. Attending a concert, opera, or ballet		
221. Playing with pets		
222. Going to a play		
223. Looking at the stars or moon		
224.		
225.		
226.		

Now, go back over the list, and, for the items you rated "2" or "1," put a check in Column S if you would find this activity pleasurable while sober.

Note. Adapted from MacPhillamy and Lewinsohn (1982).

FORM 5a COMMUNICATION SKILLS:
LEVEL I HANDOUT—EXPRESSING FEELINGS CLEARLY

Expressing your feelings clearly is an important step toward communicating effectively. The following exercise will help you get started.

"I" Message Exercise

An "I" message is a way to take responsibility for your own feelings when talking about a problem with another person. "I" messages help to identify the problem without causing the other person to be defensive. Practice using "I" messages with your partner by doing the following exercise:

1. Take a minor problem you are having with your partner. (As you become more comfortable with this skill, move on to more serious problems.)
2. Begin by saying "I have a problem," or, "I have something that I'd like to talk with you about."
3. State your concerns in the form of an "I" message, using the formula "when you _____ [behavior], I feel _____ [emotion] because _____ [specific reason]," making certain you answer the following questions:
   a. What specific behaviors is your partner doing that you have feelings about? (behavior)
   b. How do you feel about your partner's behavior? (emotion)
   c. What are the consequences the behavior has on you?
4. Request a specific change in your partner's behavior.
5. Give partner a chance to respond to your communication, including the request.
6. Reverse roles, and repeat the exercise.
7. Remember you can also use this exercise to communicate praise or pleasant feelings toward one another.

FORM 5b COMMUNICATION SKILLS:
LEVEL I HANDOUT—PERCEPTION CHECKS

A perception check is a simple yet highly effective communication technique that involves (1) identifying what you noticed, (2) stating your guess as to what that behavior means, and then (3) asking if your interpretation is accurate. The following exercise can help you practice your perception checks with each other.

Perception Checks

1. Take a recent situation (of mild disturbance) where you made an assumption about the motivations or intentions of your partner (e.g., a situation where he or she came home late and you assumed he or she forgot about your plans for the evening, or a situation where your partner didn't say "Hi" when he or she came home from work and you assumed he or she was angry). Describe the situation—just the facts—to your partner.

2. Practice the following to respond to this situation differently:
   a. Identify what you noticed (specific behavior)
   b. State your "guess" as to what this behavior indicated
   c. Ask your partner if your interpretation was accurate

3. The partner's responsibility is to clarify any misunderstandings or assumptions.

Example of Step 2:
   a. I noticed that when you came home this evening that you went directly to the bedroom and did not say "hi" to me.
   b. I felt like you were mad at me.
   c. Was my interpretation correct or was something else going on?

FORM 5c COMMUNICATION SKILLS:
LEVEL II HANDOUT—REFLECTIVE LISTENING

Reflective listening is an important, although difficult, communication skill to master. In order for the speaker to feel accepted and understood, he or she must know that the listener heard the content (information), as well as the feelings that were conveyed. As the listener, it is not important that you agree with the speakers statement, but rather that you verbalize your understanding. This style of communication may feel foreign to you at first, but with practice, can make a significant difference in your conversations.

Reflective Listening Exercise

Reflective listening means to restate, in your own words, the content and the feelings of the speaker.

1. Work with your partner. Choose a time together when you will not be interrupted.
2. Briefly write down a problem you are having with another person (other than your partner).
3. Take turns. Decide who will be first to share a problem.
4. Speaker: Briefly state the problem
5. Listener: Restate the problem and feelings accurately.
6. Speaker: Tell the listener whether or not she or he made an accurate restatement; did she or he capture the information
7. Repeat the process until the listener fully understands the speaker's concerns.

FORM 6 DRINKING CHAIN II AND FEELINGS LIST

Record in the spaces below each time you either drank or thought about drinking alcohol. Bring this chart with you to each therapy session.

DAY & TIME	SITUATION Where were you? What were you doing? Who were you with?	THOUGHTS What did you say to yourself to help make the decision?	FEELINGS See feelings list for help.	DRINK OR NOT?	RESULTS & ALTERNATIVES What happened? What else did you do or could you have done?
EXAMPLE 1: Friday 7 P.M.	Ed and Mary's house having dinner. Ed offered me wine.	I haven't had a drink in 3 weeks. Everyone else is drinking. One glass won't hurt.	Deprived, left out, then, pleased	Yes	Drank four glasses of wine. I could have had soda water instead.
EXAMPLE 2: Sunday 1 P.M.	Home alone, watching the game. Beer commercial comes on.	I usually drink beer when I watch the game but I am trying to quit.	Sorry for myself.	No	Walked around the block during the commercials. Reminded myself of commitment to abstain.

FORM 7 TARGET BEHAVIOR CHART II AND FEELINGS LIST

Behavior to reduce or eliminate: _____

Record in the spaces below each time you either engaged in or thought about engaging in the target behavior. Bring this chart with you to each therapy session.

DAY & TIME	SITUATION Where were you? What were you doing? Who were you with?	THOUGHTS What did you say to yourself to help make the decision?	FEELINGS See feelings list for help.	DRINK OR NOT?	RESULTS & ALTERNATIVES What happened? What else did you do or could you have done?
EXAMPLE 1: Friday 6 A.M.	In the kitchen, getting ready for work. Saw coffee maker. (target behavior: abstain from caffeine)	I'm really tired, and I need a cup of coffee	Tired, deprived.	Yes	I drank coffee for 2 days. I could have treated myself to a nap instead.
EXAMPLE 2: Monday 5 P.M.	Driving home from work past a new ice cream store. (target behavior: abstain from sugar)	Ice cream would taste fantastic, but I don't want to ruin my diet.	A little bit sad.	No	Didn't stop. Went home and made a healthy dinner. Called a friend to cheer myself up.

LIST OF FEELINGS (include with Forms 6 and 7)

Afraid	Secure	Distasteful
Ashamed	Strong	Exasperated
Excited	Alone	Frustrated
Hurt	Burned	Horrified
Lonely	Defeated	Joyful
Sad	Discouraged	Negative
Agonized	Jilted	Paranoid
Bashful	Tearful	Satisfied
Cautious	Bewildered	Smug
Determined	Foolish	Withdrawn
Disgusted	Impatient	Mellow
Envious	Unpopular	Respectful
Frightened	Ill at ease	Forgiving
Guilty	Jittery	Well-meaning
Hysterical	Embarrassed	Contented
Miserable	Uncomfortable	Jovial
Optimistic	Depreciated	Thrilled
Relieved	Mocked	Assured
Sheepish	Cowardly	Competent
Suspicious	Inadequate	Forceful
Loving	Aggressive	Important
Cooperative	Hostile	Powerful
Sympathetic	Angry	Self-confident
Tolerant	Desperate	Abandoned
Calm	Frustrated	Battered
Enthusiastic	Insecure	Cheapened
Serene	Remorseful	Dejected
Turned on	Worried	Gloomy
Capable	Apologetic	Left out
Fearless	Blissful	Worthless
Heroic	Confident	Clumsy
Manly	Violent	Futile

(continued)

LIST OF FEELINGS *(continued)*

Offended	Enraged	Stable
Agitated	Exhausted	Alienated
Intimidated	Grieving	Blue
Nervous	Hungover	Crushed
Scared	Mischievous	Depressed
Uneasy	Obstinate	Humiliated
Humiliated	Regretful	Mistreated
Put down	Shocked	Awkward
Demoralized	Surprised	Dissatisfied
Inferior	Affectionate	Helpless
Annoyed	Open	Tormented
Outraged	Tender	Alarmed
Anxious	Generous	Apprehensive
Disappointed	At ease	Panicky
Happy	Delighted	Shaky
Jealous	Proud	Abused
Resentful	Triumphant	Laughed at
Aggressive	Brave	Slighted
Arrogant	Determined	Impotent
Bored	Healthy	Vulnerable
Curious	Intense	Belligerent
Disapproving	Robust	Vindictive

FORM 8a RULES FOR PERSON OFFERING A DRINK/TARGET
BEHAVIOR

Use whatever maneuvers you can think of to get the other person
to give in and agree to drink or engage in the target behavior.

1. Bring up side issues.
2. Show logically why the person should accept the drink.
3. Ask questions in an attempt to throw the other person off
   balance.
4. Try to make the other person feel guilty.
5. Get angry and loud.
6. Pout.

FORM 8b RULES FOR PERSON REFUSING TO DRINK/
ENGAGE IN THE TARGET BEHAVIOR

1. Decide on one short, broken record phrase that represents how you feel or what you think about the situation (e.g., "I'm no longer drinking," or, "I don't eat sweets").
2. The first time the person offers you a drink, honestly explain why the answer is "no." Do not invent excuses. For example, don't say, "I have a stomach ache," because doing so will just postpone the situation, and you will have to continue to refuse the drink or target behavior and explain later. End your explanation with the short, broken record phrase. Do not explain your reason again. Once is enough.
3. From then on, each time the person attempts to convince you, let him or her know firmly and politely that you understand his or her feelings (argument/situation), and then end with your broken record phrase—always the EXACT, SAME broken record phrase.

Example of Refusal:

A friend says, "We've always drunk beer when we watched the Super Bowl."

You say, "I know we've always drunk beer and it was a lot of fun, but I'm no longer drinking."

Friend says, "You think you're too good for us now?"

You say, "No, it is just that I'm no longer drinking."

4. Be pleasant yet persistent and unyielding. Repeat your short statement as many times as necessary.
5. If the other person gets angry or loud, remain calm.
6. If the other person asks questions about why you are not drinking, don't answer them—this might lead you astray.
7. If the other person brings up side issues, ignore them and repeat your broken record.
8. In order to end on a friendly note, suggest an alternative, for example, "Why don't we get together next weekend for a movie instead?"

FORM 9 SUPPORT NETWORK

NAME	HOW AND WHEN I CAN COUNT ON THIS PERSON	PHONE #
Example: Bob	I can call him when I'm at a party and feel like drinking.	966-1234

FORM 10 ACTION PLAN

PRIORITY	PROBLEM AREA	GOAL	STRATEGIES	WORK ON IN SESSION #	TARGET DATE AND OUTCOME

191

FORM 11   RECOVERY PLAN

I. WHAT I LEARNED IN THE PROGRAM:

_____

_____

_____

_____

_____

_____

II. WHAT I WILL CONTINUE TO WORK ON AND HOW I WILL
     WORK ON IT (BE SPECIFIC):

_____

_____

_____

_____

_____

_____

III. HIGH-RISK SITUATIONS AND PLANS TO COPE:

_____

_____

_____

_____

_____

_____

(continued)

FORM 11   *(continued)*

IV. SUPPORT RESOURCES I WILL USE INCLUDE (INCLUDE
PHONE NUMBERS WHEN APPROPRIATE):

_____

_____

_____

_____

_____

_____

V. HOW MY PARTNER WILL SUPPORT ME (COMPLETED BY
PARTNER):

I will support you by _____

_____

_____

_____

_____

VI. OTHER HELPFUL REMINDERS:

_____

_____

_____

_____

FORM 12   CERTIFICATE OF COMPLETION

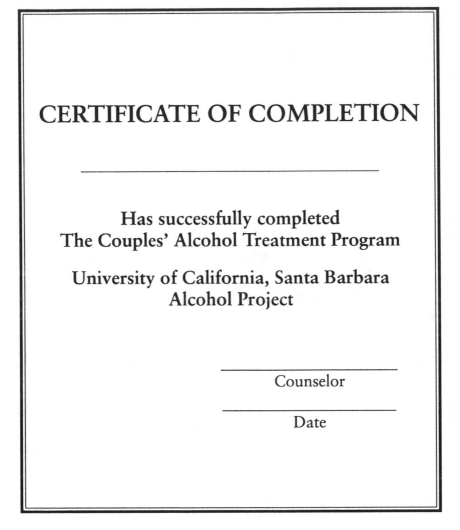

CERTIFICATE OF COMPLETION

_____

Has successfully completed
The Couples' Alcohol Treatment Program

University of California, Santa Barbara
Alcohol Project

_____
Counselor

_____
Date

References

Abel, E. L., & Sokol, R. J. (1987). Incidence of Fetal Alcohol Syndrome and economic impact of FAS-related anomalies. *Drug and Alcohol Dependence, 19,* 51–70.

Abrams, D. B. (1983). Psycho-social assessment of alcohol and stress interactions: Bridging the gap between laboratory and treatment outcome research. In L. A. Pohorecky & J. Brick (Eds.), *Stress and alcohol use* (pp. 61–86). New York: Elsevier Biomedical.

Alcoholics Anonymous. (1987). *Analysis of the membership of Alcoholics Anonymous.* New York: AA World Services, Inc., General Services Office of AA.

American Psychiatric Association. (1994). *Diagnostic and statistical manual of mental disorders* (4th ed.). Washington, DC: Author.

Bandura, A. (1977a). Self-efficacy: Toward a unifying theory of behavior change. *Psychological Review, 84,* 191–215.

Bandura, A. (1977b). *Social learning theory.* Englewood Cliffs, NJ: Prentice Hall.

Beck, A. T., Rush, A. J., Shaw, B. F., & Emery, G. (1979). *Cognitive therapy of depression.* New York: Guilford Press.

Beck, A. T., Wright, F. D., Newman, C. F., & Liese, B. S. (1993). *Cognitive therapy of substance abuse.* New York: Guilford Press.

Beckman, L. J. (1993). Alcoholics Anonymous and gender issues. In B. S. McCrady & W. R. Miller (Eds.), *Research on Alcoholics Anonymous: Opportunities and alternatives* (pp. 233–250). New Brunswick, NJ: Rutgers Center of Alcohol Studies.

Beckman, L. J., & Kocel, K. M. (1982). Treatment delivery system and alcohol abuse in women: Social policy implications. *Journal of Social Issues, 38*(2), 139–151.

Beutler, L. E., Engle, D., Mohr, D., Daldrup, R. J., Bergan, J., Meredith, K., & Merry, W. (1991). Predictors of differential response to cognitive, experiential, and self-directed psychotherapeutic procedures. *Journal of Consulting and Clinical Psychology, 59,* 333–340.

Beutler, L. E., Jovanovic, J., & Williams, R. E. (1993). Process research perspectives in Alcoholics Anonymous: Measurement of process variables. In B. S.

McCrady & W. R. Miller (Eds.), *Research on Alcoholics Anonymous: Opportunities and alternatives* (pp. 357–378). New Brunswick, NJ: Rutgers Center of Alcohol Studies.

Beutler, L. E., Williams, R. E., & Zetzer, H. A. (1994). Efficacy in the treatment of child sexual abuse. *Future of Children, 4,* 156–175.

Blume, S. (1986). Women and alcohol: A review. *Journal of the American Medical Association, 256,* 1467–1470.

Bolton, R. (1979). *People skills: How to assert yourself, listen to others, and resolve conflicts.* New York: Simon & Schuster.

Bongar, B. (1992). *Suicide: Guidelines for assessment, management, and treatment.* New York: Oxford University Press.

Brisman, J., & Siegel, M. (1984). Bulimia and alcoholics: Two sides of the same coin? *Journal of Substance Abuse Treatment, 2,* 113–118.

Burns, D. D. (1989). *The feeling good handbook.* New York: Plume.

Caetano, R. (1984). Ethnicity and drinking in Northern California: A comparison among whites, blacks and Hispanics. *Alcohol and Alcoholism, 19,* 31–44.

Caetano, R. (1986–1987). Drinking and Hispanic-American family life: The view outside the clinic walls. *Alcohol Health and Research World, 2,* 27–35.

Caetano, R. (1990). Hispanic drinking in the U.S.: Thinking in new directions. *British Journal of Addiction, 85,* 1231–1236.

Caetano, R., & Mora, M. E. M. (1988). Acculturation and drinking among people of Mexican descent in Mexico and the United States. *Journal of Studies on Alcohol, 49,* 462–471.

Caplan, G. (1974). *Support systems and community mental health: Lectures in concept development.* New York: Behavioral.

Cervantes, R. C., Gilbert, M. J., de Snyder, N. S., & Padilla, A. (1991). Psychosocial and cognitive correlates of alcohol use in younger adult immigrant and U.S.-born Hispanics. *International Journal of the Addictions, 25,* 687–708.

Chaney, E. F., O'Leary, M. R., & Marlatt, G. A. (1978). Skill training with alcoholics. *Journal of Consulting and Clinical Psychology, 46,* 1092–1104.

Chi, I., Lubben, J. E., & Kitano, H. H. L. (1989). Differences in drinking behavior among three Asian-American groups. *Journal of Studies on Alcohol, 50,* 15–23.

Corbett, K., Mora, J., & Ames, G. (1991). Drinking patterns and drinking-related problems of Mexican-American husbands and wives. *Journal of Studies on Alcohol, 52,* 215–223.

Cummings, C., Gordon, J., & Marlatt, G. A. (1980). Relapse: Strategies of prevention and prediction. In W. R. Miller (Ed.), The addictive behaviors (pp. 291–321). Oxford, United Kingdom: Pergamon Press.

Dunne, F. (1988). Are women more easily damaged by alcohol than men? *British Journal of Addiction, 83*(10), 1135–1136.

Frieze, I. H., & Schaefer, P. C. (1984). Alcohol use and marital violence: Female and male differences in reactions to alcohol. In S. C. Wilsnack & L. J. Beckman (Eds.), *Alcohol problems in women: Antecedents, consequences, and intervention* (pp. 260–279). New York: Guilford Press.

Geller, A. (1991a). *Restore your life: A living plan for sober people.* New York: Bantam.

Geller, A. (1991b). The effects of drug use during pregnancy. In P. Roth (Ed.), *Alcohol and drugs are women's issues: Vol. 1. A review of the issues* (pp. 101–106). Metuchen, NJ: Women's Action Alliance & Scarecrow Press.

Gomberg, E. S. L. (1987). Shame and guilt issues among women alcoholics. Alcoholism Treatment Quarterly, 4(2), 139–155.

Gomberg, E. S. (1974). Women and alcoholism. In V. Frank & V. Burtle (Eds.), *Women in therapy* (pp. 169–190). New York: Brunner/Mazel.

Gomberg, E. S. (1981). Women, sex roles, and alcohol problems. *Professional Psychology, 12*(1), 146–155.

Gomberg, E. S. L. (1989). Suicide risk among women with alcohol problems. *American Journal of Public Health, 79,* 1363–1365.

Gondoli, D. M., & Jacob, T. (1990). Family treatment of alcoholism. In R. R. Watson (Ed.), *Drug and alcohol abuse prevention* (pp. 245–262). New York: Humana Press.

Gordon, A. J., & Zrull, M. (1991). Social networks and recovery: One year after inpatient treatment. *Journal of Substance Abuse Treatment, 8,* 143–152.

Gorski, T. T. (1989). *Passages through recovery: An action plan for preventing relapse.* Center City, NM: Hazelden Educational Materials.

Hammer, T., & Vaglum, P. (1989). The increase in alcohol consumption among women: A phenomenon related to accessibility or stress? A general population study. *British Journal of Addiction, 84,* 767–775.

Harlap, S., & Shiono, P. H. (1980). Alcohol, smoking, and incidence of spontaneous abortions in first and second trimester. *Lancet, 2,* 173–176.

Harper, F. D. (1984). Group strategies with black alcoholics. *Journal for the Specialists in Group Work, 9,* 38–43.

Helzer, J. E., & Pryzbeck, T. R. (1988). The co-occurrence of alcoholism with other psychiatric disorders in the general population with its impact on treatment. *Journal of Studies on Alcohol, 49,* 219–224.

Henzel, H. A. (1984). Diagnosing alcoholism in patients with anorexia nervosa. *American Journal of Drug and Alcohol Abuse, 10,* 461–466.

Herd, D. (1989). The epidemiology of drinking patterns and alcohol-related problems among U.S. Blacks. In L. Speigler, D. A. Tate, S. Aiken, & M. Christian (Eds.), *Alcohol use among U.S. ethnic minorities* (NIAAA Research Monograph 18, DHHS Publication No. ADM 89-1435, pp. 3–50). Rockville, MD: U.S. Department of Health and Human Services.

Hesselbrock, M. N., & Hesselbrock, V. M. (1993). Depression and antisocial personality disorder in alcoholism: Gender comparison. In E. S. L. Gomberg & T. D. Nirenberg (Eds.), *Women and substance abuse* (pp. 142–161). Norwood, NJ: Ablex.

Hesselbrock, M. N., Hesselbrock, V. M., Syzmanski, K., & Weidenman, M. A. (1988). Suicide attempts and alcoholism. *Journal of Studies on Alcohol, 49,* 436–442.

Hesselbrock, M. N., Meyer, R. E., & Keener, J. (1985). Psychopathology in hospitalized alcoholics. *Archives of General Psychiatry, 42,* 1050–1055.

Hill, S. Y. (1984). Vulnerability to the biomedical consequences of alcoholism and alcohol-related problems among women. In S. C. Wilsnack & L. J. Beckman

(Eds.), *Alcohol problems in women: Antecedents, consequences, and intervention* (pp. 121–154). New York: Guilford Press.

Hilton, M. E. (1987). Drinking patterns and drinking problems in 1984: Results from a general population survey. *Alcoholism: Clinical and Experimental Research, 11*(2), 167–175.

Holck, S., Warren, C., Smith, J., & Rochat, W. (1984). Alcohol consumption among Mexican American and Anglo women: Results of survey along the U. S. Mexican border. *Journal of Studies on Alcohol, 45,* 149–154.

Hurley, D. L. (1991). Women, alcohol and incest: An analytical review. *Journal of Studies on Alcohol, 52,* 253–268.

Institute of Medicine. (1990). *Broadening the base of treatment for alcohol problems.* Washington, DC: National Academy Press.

Jacob, T., & Bremer, D. A. (1986). Assortative mating among men and women alcoholics. *Journal of Studies on Alcohol, 47,* 219–222.

Jacobson, N. E., Holtzworth-Munroe, A., & Schmaling, K. B. (1989). Martial therapy and spouse involvement in the treatment of depression, agoraphobia, and alcoholism. *Journal of Consulting and Clinical Psychology, 57,* 5–10.

Johnson, S. (1991). Recent research: Alcohol and women's bodies. In P. Roth (Ed.), *Alcohol and drugs are women's issues: Vol. 1. A review of the issues* (pp. 32–42). Metuchen, NJ: Women's Action Alliance & Scarecrow Press.

Jones, B. M., & Jones, M. K. (1976). Women and alcohol: Intoxication, metabolism, and the menstrual cycle. In M. Greenblatt & M. Schuckit (Eds.), *Alcohol problems in women and children* (pp. 103–136). New York: Grune & Stratton.

Jones, M. K., & Jones, B. M. (1984). Ethanol metabolism in women taking oral contraceptives. *Alcoholism: Clinical and Experimental Research, 8*(1), 24–28.

Kadden, R., Carroll, K., Donovan, D., Cooney, N., Monti, P., Abrams, D., Litt, M., & Hester, R. (1989). *Cognitive- behavioral coping skill therapy manual. A clinical research guide for therapists treating individuals with alcohol abuse and dependence.* Rockville, MD: U.S. Department of Health and Human Services.

Kline, J., Shrout, R., Stein, Z., Susser, M., & Warburton, D. (1980). Drinking during pregnancy and spontaneous abortion. *Lancet, 2,* 176–180.

Krahn, D. D. (1993). The relationship of eating disorders and substance abuse. In E. S. L. Gomberg & T. D. Nirenberg (Eds.), *Women and substance abuse* (pp. 286–313). Norwood, NJ: Ablex.

LaDue, R. A. (1991). Coyote returns: Survival for Native American women. In P. Roth (Ed.), *Alcohol and drugs are women's issues: Vol. 1. A review of the issues* (pp. 23– 31). Metuchen, NJ: Women's Action Alliance & Scarecrow Press.

Lazarus, R. S., & Folkman, S. (1984). *Stress, appraisal and coping.* New York: Springer.

Lemert, E. (1982). Drinking among American Indians. In E. L. Gomberg, H. R. White, & J. Carpenter (Eds.), *Alcohol, science and society, revisited* (pp. 80–95). New Brunswick, NJ: Rutgers Center of Alcohol Studies.

Lieber, C. S. (1993). Women and alcohol: Gender differences in metabolism and susceptibility. In E. S. L. Gomberg & T. D. Nirenberg (Eds.), *Women and substance abuse* (pp. 1–17). Norwood, NJ: Ablex.

Liepman, M. R., Goldman, R. E., Monroe, A. D., Green, K. W., Sattler, A. L., Broadhurst, J. B., & Gomberg, E. S. L. (Eds.). (1993). Substance abuse by special populations of women. In E. S. L. Gomberg & T. D. Nirenberg (Eds.), *Women and substance abuse* (pp. 214–257). Norwood, NJ: Ablex.

Lillie-Blanton, M., Mackenzie, E., & Anthony, J. (1991). Black–white differences in alcohol use by women: Baltimore survey findings. *Public Health Reports, 10*, 124–133.

Little, R. E., & Ervin, C. H. (1984). Alcohol use and reproduction. In S. C. Wilsnack & L. J. Beckman (Eds.), *Alcohol problems in women: Antecedents, consequences, and intervention* (pp. 155–188). New York: Guilford Press.

Little, R. E., & Wendt, J. K. (1993). The effects of maternal drinking in the reproductive period: An epidemiological review. In E. S. L. Gomberg & T. D. Nirenberg (Eds.), *Women and substance abuse* (pp. 191–209). Norwood, NJ: Ablex.

Longabaugh, R., Beattie, M., Stout, R., Malloy, P., & Noel, N. (1988, February). *Environmental treatment of alcohol abusers.* Paper presented at Evaluating Recovery Outcomes Conference, University of California at San Diego.

Longnecker, M. P., Berlin, J. A., Orza, M. J., & Chalmers, T. C. (1988). A meta-analysis of alcohol consumption in relation to risk of breast cancer. *Journal of the American Medical Association, 260*, 652–656.

Lowenfels, A. B., & Zevola, S. A. (1989). Alcohol and breast cancer: An overview. *Alcoholism: Clinical and Experimental Research, 13*, 109–111.

Lutz, M. E. (1991). Sobering decisions: Are there gender differences? *Alcoholism Treatment Quarterly, 8*(2), 51–65.

MacPhillamy, D. J., & Lewinsohn, P. M. (1982). The Pleasant Events Scale: Studies on reliability, validity, and scale intercorrelations. *Journal of Consulting and Clinical Psychology, 50*(3), 363–380.

Marlatt, G. A., & Gordon, J. R. (Eds.). (1985). *Relapse prevention: Maintenance strategies in the treatment of addictive behaviors.* New York: Guilford Press.

May, P. A., & Hymbaugh, K. J. (1983). A pilot project on Fetal Alcohol Syndrome among American Indians. *Alcohol Health and Research World, 7*, 3–9.

McCarthy, B. W. (1992). Erectile dysfunction and inhibited sexual desire: Cognitive-behavioral strategies. *Journal of Sex Education and Therapy, 18*(1), 22–34.

McCrady, B. S. (1982). Conjoint behavior treatment of an alcoholic and his spouse: The case of Mr. and Mrs. D.. In W. Hay & P. Nathan (Eds.), *Clinical case studies in the behavior treatment of alcoholism* (pp. 127–156). New York: Plenum.

McCrady, B. S. (1989). Extending relapse prevention models to couples. *Addictive Behaviors, 14*, 69–74.

McCrady, B. S., Dean, L., Dubreuil, E., & Swanson, S. (1985). The Problem Drinkers' Project: A programmatic application of social-learning-based treatment. In G. A. Marlatt & J. R. Gordon (Eds.), *Relapse prevention: Maintenance strategies in the treatment of addictive behaviors* (pp. 417–471). New York: Guilford Press.

McCrady, B. S., Noel, N. E., Abrams, D. B., Stout, R. L., Nelson, H. F., & Hay, W. H. (1986). Comparative effectiveness of three types of spouse involvement in outpatient behavioral alcoholism outpatient treatment. *Journal of Studies on Alcohol, 47,* 459–467.

McCrady, B. S., & Raytek, H. (1993). Women and substance abuse: Treatment modalities and outcomes. In E. S. L. Gomberg & T. D. Nirenberg (Eds.), *Women and substance abuse* (pp. 314– 338). Norwood, NJ: Ablex.

McCrady, B. S., & Smith, D. E. (1986). Implications of cognitive impairment for the treatment of alcoholism. *Alcoholism: Clinical and Experimental Research, 10,* 145–149.

McMullin, R. E. (1986). *Handbook of cognitive therapy techniques.* New York: W. W. Norton.

Miller, B. A. (1990). The interrelationships between alcohol and drugs and family violence. *National Institute on Drug Abuse Research Monograph Series, 103,* 177–207.

Miller, B. A., Downs, W. R., & Gondoli, D. M. (1989). Spousal violence among alcoholic women as compared to a random household sample of women. *Journal of Studies on Alcohol, 50*(6), 533–540.

Miller, W. R., & Hester, R. K. (1986). Inpatient alcohol treatment: Who benefits? *American Psychologist, 41,* 794–805.

Monti, P. M., Abrams, D. B., Kadden, R. M., & Cooney, N. L. (1989). *Treating alcohol dependence: A coping skills training guide.* New York: Guilford Press.

Mora, J., & Gilbert, M. J. (1991). Issues for Latinas: Mexican American women. In P. Roth. (Ed.), *Alcohol and drugs are women's issues: Vol 1. A review of the issues* (pp. 43–47). Metuchen, NJ: Women's Action Alliance & Scarecrow Press.

Morgenstern, J., & McCrady, B. S. (1992). Curative factors in alcohol and drug treatment: Behavioral and disease model perspectives. *British Journal of Addiction, 87,* 901–912.

Nathan, P. E. (1986). Outcomes of treatment for alcoholism: Current data. *Annals of Behavioral Medicine, 8,* 40–46.

National Institute on Drug Abuse. (1990). *Highlights from the 1989 National Drug and Alcoholism Treatment Survey (NDATUS).* Rockville, MD: Author.

Noel, N. E., McCrady, B. S., Stout, R. L., & Fisher-Nelson, H. (1991). Gender differences in marital functioning of male and female alcoholics. *Family Dynamics of Addiction Quarterly, 1*(4), 31–38.

O'Farrell, T. J. (1989). Marital and family therapy in alcoholism treatment. *Journal of Substance Abuse Treatment, 6,* 23–29.

O'Farrell, T. J. (1991). Using couples therapy in the treatment of alcoholism. *Family Dynamics in Addiction Quarterly, 1,* 39–45.

O'Farrell, T. J. (Ed.). (1993). *Treating alcohol problems: Marital and family interventions.* New York: Guilford Press.

O'Farrell, T. J., & Bayog, R. D. (1986). Antabuse contracts for married alcoholics and their spouses: A method to maintain antabuse ingestion and decrease conflict about drinking. *Journal of Substance Abuse Treatment, 3,* 1–8.

O'Farrell, T. J., Cutter, H. S. G., Choquette, F. J., & Bayog, R. D. (1992). Behavioral marital therapy for male alcoholics: Marital and drinking adjustment during the two years after treatment. *Behavior Therapy, 23,* 529–549.

O'Farrell, T. J., & Murphy, C. M. (1995). Marital violence before and after alcoholism treatment. *Journal of Consulting and Clinical Psychology, 63*(2), 256–262.

Oyabu, N., & Garland, T. N. (1987). An investigation of the impact of social support on the outcome of an alcoholism treatment program. *International Journal of the Addictions, 22*(3), 221–234.

Palfai, T., & Jankiewicz, H. (1991). *Drugs and human behavior.* Dubuque, IA: Wm. C. Brown Publishers.

Perodeau, G. M. (1984). Married alcoholic women: A review. *Journal of Drug Issues, 14,* 703–719.

Peveler, R., & Fairburn, C. (1990). Eating disorders in women who abuse alcohol. *British Journal of Addiction, 85,* 1633–1638.

Piazza, N. J., Vrbka, J. L., & Yeager, R. D. (1989). Telescoping of alcoholism in women alcoholics. *International Journal of the Addictions, 24*(1), 19–28.

Prochaska, J. O., DiClemente, C. C., & Norcross, J. C. (1992). In search of how people change: Applications to addictive behaviors. *American Psychologist, 47*(9), 1102–1114.

Robbins, C. (1989). Sex differences in psychosocial consequences of alcohol and drug use. *Journal of Health and Social Behavior, 30,* 117–130.

Rohsenow, D. J., Corbett, R., & Devine, D. (1988). Molested as children: A hidden contribution to substance abuse? *Journal of Substance Abuse Treatment, 5,* 13–18.

Roman, P. M. (1988). Treatment issues. In *Women and alcohol use: A review of the research literature* (NIAAA, DHHS Publication No. ADM 88-1574). Rockville, MD: U.S. Department of Health and Human Services.

Ronan, L. (1986–1987). Alcohol-related health risks among Black Americans. *Alcohol Health and Research World,* 36–39.

Rosenberg, H. (1993). Prediction of controlled drinking by alcoholics and problem drinkers. *Psychological Bulletin, 113,* 129–139.

Roth, P. (Ed.). (1991). *Alcohol and drugs are women's issues: Vol. 1. A review of the issues.* Metuchen, NJ: Women's Action Alliance & Scarecrow Press.

Russell, M. (1989). Alcohol use and related problems among black and white gynecologic patients. In L. Speigler, D. A. Tate, S. Aiken, & M. Christian (Eds.), *Alcohol use among U.S. ethnic minorities* (NIAAA Research Monograph 18, DHHS Publication No. ADM 89-1435, pp. 77–94). Rockville, MD: U.S. Department of Health and Human Services.

Russell, S. A., & Wilsnack, S. C. (1991). Adult survivors of childhood sexual abuse: Substance abuse and other consequences. In P. Roth (Ed.), *Alcohol and drugs are women's issues: Vol. 1. A review of the issues* (pp. 61–70). Metuchen, NJ: Women's Action Alliance & Scarecrow Press.

Schaefer, S., & Evans, S. (1987). Women, sexuality, and the process of recovery. *Journal of Chemical Dependency Treatment, 1,* 91–120.

Schlesinger, S., Susman, M., & Koenigsberg, J. (1990). Self-esteem and purpose in life: A comparative study of women alcoholics. *Journal of Alcohol and Drug Education, 36*(1), 127–141.

Schmidt, C., Klee, L., & Ames, G. (1990). Review and analysis of literature on indicators of women's drinking problems. *British Journal of Addiction, 85,* 179–192.

Schuckit, M. A., & Monteiro, M. G. (1988). Alcoholism, anxiety, and depression. *British Journal of Addiction, 83,* 1373–1380.

Smith, L. (1992). Help seeking in alcohol-dependent females. *Alcohol and Alcoholism, 27*(1), 3–9.

Smith, M. J. (1975). *When I say no, I feel guilty.* New York: Dial Press.

Sobell, M. B., & Sobell, L. C. (1993). *Problem drinkers: Guided self-change treatment.* New York: Guilford Press.

Taha-Cisse, A. H. (1991). Issues for African-American women. In P. Roth (Ed.), *Alcohol and drugs are women's issues: Vol. 1. A review of the issues* (pp. 54–60). Metuchen, NJ: Women's Action Alliance & Scarecrow Press.

Taysi, K. (1988). Preconceptual counseling. *Obstetrics and Gynecology Clinics of North America, 15,* 167–178.

Tiefer, L., & Melman, A. (1989). Comprehensive evaluation of erectile dysfunction and medical treatments. In S. R. Leiblum & R. C. Rosen (Eds.), *Principles and practice of sex therapy: Update for the 1990s* (2nd ed., pp. 207–236). New York: Guilford Press.

Turnbull, J. E., & Gomberg, E. S. L. (1988). Impact of depressive symptomatology on alcohol problems in women. *Alcoholism: Clinical and Experimental Research, 12,* 374–381.

Urban, H. B., & Ford, D. H. (1971). Some historical and conceptual perspectives on psychotherapy and behavior change. In S. L. Bergin & A. E. Garfield (Eds.), *Handbook of psychotherapy and behavior change: An empirical analysis* (p. 8) New York: Wiley.

Vannicelli, M. (1984). Treatment outcome of alcoholic women: The state of the art in relation to sex bias and expectancy effects. In S. C. Wilsnack & L. J. Beckman (Eds.), *Alcohol problems in women: Antecedents, consequences, and intervention* (pp. 369–412). New York: Guilford Press.

Vannicelli, M., & Nash, L. (1984). Effect of bias on women's studies on alcoholism. *Alcoholism: Clinical and Experimental Research, 8,* 334–336.

Wilsnack, R. W., & Cheloha, R. (1987). Women's roles and problem drinking across the lifespan. *Social Problems, 34*(3), 231–248.

Wilsnack, R. W., Wilsnack, S. C., & Klassen, A. D. (1984). Women's drinking and drinking problems: Patterns from a 1981 national survey. *American Journal of Public Health, 74*(11), 1231–1238.

Wilsnack, S. C. (1991). Sexuality and women's drinking: Findings from a U.S. national study. *Special Issue: Alcohol and Sexuality. Alcohol, Health and the Research World, 15,* 147–150.

Wilsnack, S. C., & Beckman, L. J. (Eds.). (1984). *Alcohol problems in women: Antecedents, consequences, and intervention.* New York: Guilford Press.

Wilsnack, S. C., Klassen, A. D., & Wilsnack, R. W. (1984). Drinking and reproductive dysfunction among women in a 1981 national survey. *Alcoholism: Clinical and Experimental Research, 8,* 451–458.

Wilsnack, S. C., & Wilsnack, R. W. (1993). Epidemiological research on women's drinking: Recent progress and directions for the 1990s. In E. S. L. Gomberg and T. D. Nirenberg (Eds.), *Women and substance abuse* (pp. 62–99). Norwood, NJ: Ablex.

Wilsnack, S. C., Wilsnack, R. W., & Klassen, A. D. (1986). Epidemiological research on women's drinking, 1978–1984. In *Women and alcohol: Health-related issues* (NIAAA Research Monograph 16, DHHS Publication No. ADM 86-1139, pp. 1–68). Washington, DC: U.S. Government Printing Office.

Wilson, G. T. (1989). Behavior therapy. In R. J. Corsini & D. Wedding (Eds.), *Current psychotherapies* (4th ed., pp. 241–282). Itasca, IL: Peacock.

Windle, M., & Miller, B. A. (1989). Alcoholism and depressive symptomatology among convicted DWI men and women. *Journal of Studies on Alcohol, 50,* 406–413.

Index